ABC OF
PSYCHOLOGICAL MEDICINE

ABC OF
PSYCHOLOGICAL MEDICINE

Edited by

RICHARD MAYOU

Professor of Psychiatry, University of Oxford, Warneford Hospital, Oxford

MICHAEL SHARPE

Reader in Psychological Medicine, University of Edinburgh

and

ALAN CARSON

*Consultant Neuropsychiatrist, NHS Lothian and Honorary Senior Lecturer,
University of Edinburgh*

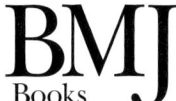

First published in 2003

by BMJ Books, BMA House, Tavistock Square,
London WC1H 9JR

www.bmjbooks.com

British Library Cataloguing in Publication Data
A catalogue record for this book is available from the British Library

ISBN 0 7279 1556 8

Typeset by Newgen Imaging Systems and BMJ Electronic Production
Printed and bound in Spain by GraphyCems, Navarra

Cover image depicts computer artwork of a face patterned with vertical lines with a magnetic
resonance imaging (MRI) scan in the background. The MRI scan allows the internal features of
the head to be seen. At the centre is the nasal cavity (red), and above that is the front part
of the brain (blue and red). This region of the brain is part of the cerebrum, and is concerned
with conscious thought, personality and memory. With permission from
Alfred Pasieka/Science Photo Library.

Contents

Contributors

Christopher Bass
Consultant, Department of Psychological Medicine,
John Radcliffe Hospital, Oxford

Michael Boyle
General Practitioner, Linlithgow Health Centre, Linlithgow,
West Lothian

Tom Brown
Consultant Psychiatrist, St John's Hospital at Howden,
Livingston, West Lothian

Alan Carson
Consultant Neuropsychiatrist, NHS Lothian and Honorary
Senior Lecturer, University of Edinburgh

Andrew Farmer
Senior Research Fellow, Department of Public Health and
Primary Care, University of Oxford

Linda Gask
Reader in Psychiatry, University of Manchester

Russell E Glasgow
Senior Scientist, AMC Cancer Research Center, Denver,
Colorado, USA

Elspeth Guthrie
Professor of Psychological Medicine and Medical Psychotherapy,
School of Psychiatry and Behavioural Sciences, University of
Manchester

Allan House
Professor of Liaison Psychiatry, Academic Unit of Psychiatry and
Behavioural Sciences, School of Medicine, University of Leeds

Michael Von Korff
Senior Investigator, Center for Health Studies, Group Health
Cooperative of Puget Sound, Seattle, WA, USA

Laurence Leaver
General Practitioner, Jericho Health Centre, Oxford

Una Macleod
Lecturer in General Practice, Department of General Practice,
University of Glasgow

Chris J Main
Head of the Department of Behavioural Medicine, Hope
Hospital, Salford

Stephanie May
General Practitioner, Stockwell Group Practice,
Stockwell Road, London

Richard Mayou
Professor of Psychiatry, University of Oxford,
Warneford Hospital, Oxford

Robert Peveler
Professor of Liaison Psychiatry, University of Southampton

Jonathan Price
Clinical Tutor in Psychiatry, Department of Psychiatry,
University of Oxford

Gary Rodin
Professor of Psychiatry, University of Toronto, Canada

Michael Sharpe
Reader in Psychological Medicine,
University of Edinburgh

Dan Stark
Specialist Regsitrar in Medical Oncology,
Academic Unit of Oncology, St James's University Hospital,
Leeds

David Thompson
Professor of Medicine, Section of Gastrointestinal Science,
Hope Hospital, Salford

Tim Usherwood
Professor in General Practice, University of Sydney,
NSW, Australia

Craig A White
Macmillan Consultant in Psychosocial Oncology,
Ayrshire and Arran Primary Care NHS Trust

David Wilks
Consultant in Infectious Diseases, Western General Hospital,
Edinburgh

Amanda C de C Williams
Senior Lecturer in Clinical Health Psychology,
Guy's, King's, and St Thomas's School of Medicine,
University of London

Preface

Psychological medicine has a long history. Until the development of pharmacological and other specific treatments, it was a mainstay of a physician's practice. Since then the successes of biomedical theory during the 20th century have led to a loss of interest in the psychological aspects of medicine and core clinical skills have sometimes been neglected. Although many modern doctors are comfortable with the latest advances in molecular medicine, they lack confidence in applying similar intellectual rigour to the psychological problems of their patients. These deficiencies are particularly apparent in the management of patients with chronic disease and of patients whose symptoms seem out of proportion to disease pathology.

Accumulating research evidence now clearly shows that psychological variables make a substantial contribution to the outcome of most common medical conditions. The identification of problems, appropriate formulation and the implementation of appropriate treatment results in not only better outcomes for patients but also in greater satisfaction for the doctors treating them. A rediscovery of the psychological aspects of medicine is underway.

This *ABC of psychological medicine* is a practical and evidence based overview of the psychological aspects of medical practice. It aims to guide practitioners and to provide them with not only relevant information but also an intellectual structure for assessing and managing their patients. The emphasis is on day to day practice and problems rather than psychological theory. The book assumes knowledge of medical assessment, investigation, and treatment.

The opening three chapters describe general principles within which individual assessment and treatment can be formulated. They include the clinical examination and the initiation of treatment but also a critique of the structure within which care is delivered, which can often be as critical as the individual's consultation. The following three chapters describe the core skills of psychological medicine: the assessment and management of anxiety, depression, and functional somatic symptoms. The remaining chapters then describe how these skills are transferred and adapted in specific situations including the care of patients with cancer, trauma, musculoskeletal pain, fatigue, chest pain, abdominal pain, and delirium. This list is not comprehensive but provides a range of examples that should help the reader to adapt the principles to their own practice.

Psychological medicine is an extension of existing clinical knowledge and skills. Indeed many practitioners will recognise it as a formalisation of the medicine they have been practising for many years. We hope that this book will both engage the curiosity and interest of those to whom the subject matter is novel, and encourage and inform those who already understand and apply its principles.

Richard Mayou, Michael Sharpe, Alan J Carson, 2002

Introduction

It is becoming increasingly clear that we can improve medical care by paying more attention to psychological aspects of medical assessment and treatment. The study and practice of such factors is often called psychological medicine. Although the development of specialist consultation-liaison psychiatry (liaison psychiatry in the United Kingdom) and health psychology contribute to psychological medicine, the task is much wider and has major implications for the organisation and practice of care. This book aims to explain some of those implications.

Disorders that are traditionally, and perhaps misleadingly, termed "psychiatric" are highly prevalent in medical populations. At least 25-30% of general medical patients have coexisting depressive, anxiety, somatoform, or alcohol misuse disorders.[1] Several factors account for the co-occurrence of medical and psychiatric disorders. First, a medical disorder can occasionally be a cause of the psychiatric disorder (for example, hypothyroidism as a biological cause of depression). Second, cardiovascular diseases, neurological disorders, cancer, diabetes, and many other medical diseases increase the risk of depression and other psychiatric disorders. Such so called comorbidity is common, but its causal linkage with psychological conditions remains poorly understood. A third factor is coincidence—common conditions such as hypertension and depression may coexist in the same patient because both are prevalent.

Another reason for psychological medicine is the prevalence of symptoms that are unexplained by disease. Although physical symptoms account for more than half of all visits to doctors, at least a third of these symptoms remain medically unexplained.[2,3] This phenomenon is referred to as somatisation—the seeking of health care for somatic symptoms that suggest a medical disorder but represent instead an underlying depressive, anxiety, or somatoform disorder. Most patients with these mental disorders preferentially report somatic rather than emotional symptoms. Further, there are the common but poorly understood symptom syndromes such as fibromyalgia, irritable bowel syndrome, and chronic fatigue syndrome, for which the relative contributions of mind and body are not yet elucidated.[4]

Psychological medicine is important in the management of all these problems; both psychotropic medications and cognitive behavioural treatments have proved effective in the treatment of common physical symptoms and syndromes in numerous studies in general practice.[5,6] Although such treatments have traditionally been considered "psychiatric", they are also beneficial in patients without overt psychiatric disorders. Countries on both sides of the Atlantic have a long way to go in developing psychological medicine, the chasm in America between medical and psychiatric care is particularly deep. The "carve out" or organisational separations of mental health services in the managed care systems in the United States is one example of how ingrained the dualism of mind and body still is and of the reconciliation that must occur.

Psychological medicine does not mean relabelling all such patients as "psychiatric". Many patients prefer to have these problems regarded as "medical" and conceptualised in terms of a neurotransmitter imbalance or a functional bodily disturbance.[7] Concomitant psychological distress is best framed in terms of being a consequence rather than a cause of persistent physical symptoms. Premature efforts to reattribute somatic complaints to psychological mechanisms may be perceived by the patient as rejection. A more aetiologically neutral but psychologically sophisticated approach that initially focuses on symptomatic treatment, reassurance, activation, and restoration of function has proved more effective.[8]

There are better alternatives than simply to relegate such problems to the province of specialist psychiatry. One is to train general practitioners to diagnose and treat common "psychiatric" disorders.[9] Although treatment with psychotropic medication is their most feasible option, general practitioners can also be trained to deliver other psychological treatments. A second option is to use nurses or social workers with specialised training who can work with general practitioners or psychiatrists to manage medication as well as deliver psychotherapies and behavioural interventions. A third model is collaborative care, where the general practitioner's management is augmented but not replaced by visits to a psychiatrist, often on site in the general practitioner's surgery. Stepped care provides an overall principle of management whereby patients only move on to more complex and expensive forms of care where simpler management by the healthcare team is either ineffective or inappropriate. Most studies have been conducted in general medical practices, but patients seen by medical specialists also warrant attention.[3]

Psychological medicine may also be delivered in innovative ways. Promising data exist for behavioural interventions conducted outside the doctor's office, including case management by telephone, cognitive behavioural therapy given through a computer, bibliotherapy—self study by patients—and home visits (for example, for chronic fatigue syndrome).

Medical treatment that integrates a psychological approach has been shown to improve patient outcomes. The benefits of treating common physical symptoms and psychological distress effectively in medical patients include not only improved quality of life and social and work functioning, but also greater satisfaction on the part of patient and doctor and reduced use of healthcare services.[2]

What do we need to do? Better detection of these problems need not be time consuming. For example, screening for depression may require as few as one or two questions. Optimal management of patients with persistent physical symptoms and common mental disorders may require longer or more frequent visits to a doctor, help in educating and following up patients by a nurse case manager, other system changes, and specialist mental health consultations for more complex cases.[10] The competing demands of general practice must be explicitly addressed if we are to enable the general practitioner to practise psychological medicine effectively.[11]

Yet this approach is no different to what is also required for many chronic medical disorders such as diabetes, asthma, and heart disease, for which it has been proved that care in concordance with guidelines requires appreciable reorganisation of medical services.[12]

Neither chronic "medical" nor "psychiatric" disorders can be managed adequately in the current environment of general practice, where the typical patient must be seen in 10–15 minutes or less. The quick visit may work for the patient with a common cold or a single condition, such as well controlled hypertension, but will not suffice for the prevalent and disabling symptoms and disorders comprising psychological medicine. Evidence based treatments exist. Using them in a way that is integrated with general medical care will improve both patients' physical health and their psychological wellbeing.

Kurt Kroenke*
Professor of Medicine, Department of Medicine,
Regenstrief Institute for Health Care,
Indianapolis, IN, USA

* KK has received fees for speaking and research from Pfizer and Eli Lilly.

References

1. Ormel J, Von Korff M, Ustun TB, Pini S, Korten A, Oldehinkel T. Common mental disorders and disability across cultures: results from the WHO collaborative study on psychological problems in general health care. *JAMA* 1994;272:1741-48.
2. Kroenke K. Studying symptoms: sampling and measurement issues. *Ann Intern Med* 2001;134:844-55.
3. Reid S, Wessely S, Crayford T, Hotopf M. Medically unexplained symptoms in frequent attenders of secondary health care: retrospective cohort study. *BMJ* 2001;322:1-4.
4. Wessely S, Nimnuan C, Sharpe M. Functional somatic syndromes: one or many? *Lancet* 1999;354:936-9.
5. O'Malley PG, Jackson JL, Santoro J, Tomkins G, Balden E, Kroenke K. Antidepressant therapy for unexplained symptoms and symptom syndromes. *J Fam Pract* 1999;48:980-90.
6. Kroenke K, Swindle R. Cognitive-behavioral therapy for somatization and symptom syndromes: a critical review of controlled clinical trials. *Psychother Psychosom* 2000;69:205-15.
7. Sharpe M, Carson A. "Unexplained"somatic symptoms, functional syndromes, and somatization: do we need a paradigm shift? *Ann Intern Med* 2001;134:926-30.
8. Von Korff M, Moore JC. Stepped care for back pain: activating approaches for primary care. *Ann Intern Med* 2001;134:911-17.
9. Kroenke K, Taylor-Vaisey A, Dietrich AJ, Oxman TE. Interventions to improve provider diagnosis and treatment of mental disorders in primary care: a critical review of the literature. *Psychosomatics* 2000;41:39-52.
10. Rubenstein LV, Jackson-Triche M, Unutzer J, Miranda J, Minnium K, Pearson ML, et al. Evidence-based care for depression in managed primary care practices. *Health Aff* 1999;18:89-105.
11. Klinkman MS. Competing demands in psychosocial care: a model for the identification and treatment of depressive disorders in primary care. *Gen Hosp Psychiatry* 1997;19:98-111.
12. Wagner EH, Austin BT, Von Korff M. Organizing care for patients with chronic illness. *Milbank Q* 1996;74:511-44.

1   The consultation

Linda Gask, Tim Usherwood

The success of any consultation depends on how well the patient and doctor communicate with each other. There is now firm evidence linking the quality of this communication to clinical outcomes.

The dual focus—Patients are not exclusively physically ill or exclusively emotionally distressed. Often they are both. At the start of a consultation it is usually not possible to distinguish between these states. It is the doctor's task to listen actively to the patient's story, seeking and noticing evidence for both physical illness and emotional distress.

Involving patients—Changes in society and health care in the past decade have resulted in real changes in what people expect from their doctors and in how doctors view patients. In addition, greater emphasis has been placed on the reduction of risk factors, with attempts to persuade people to take preventive action and avoid risks to health. Many patients want more information than they are given. They also want to take some part in deciding about their treatment in the light of its chances of success and any side effects. Some patients, of course, do not wish to participate in decision making; they would prefer their doctor to decide on a single course of action and to advise them accordingly. The skill lies in achieving the correct balance for each patient.

A comprehensive model—The "three function" model for the medical encounter provides a template for the parallel functions of the clinical interview. This is now widely used in medical schools.

Starting the interview

Research has shown the importance of listening to patients' opening statements without interruption. Doctors often ask about the first issue mentioned by their patients, yet this may not be what is concerning them most. Once a doctor has interrupted, patients rarely introduce new issues. If uninterrupted, most patients stop talking within 60 seconds, often well before. The doctor can then ask if a patient has any further concerns, summarise what the patient has just said, or propose an agenda—"I wonder if I could start by asking you some more questions about your headaches, then we need to discuss the worries that your son has been causing you."

Detecting and responding to emotional issues

Even when their problems are psychological or social, patients usually present with physical symptoms. They are also likely to give verbal or non-verbal cues. Verbal cues are words or phrases that hint at psychological or social problems. Non-verbal cues include changes in posture, eye contact, and tone of voice that reflect emotional distress.

It is important to notice and respond to cues at the time they are offered by patients. Failure to do so may inhibit patients from further disclosures and limit the consultation to discussion of physical symptoms. Conversely, physical symptoms must be taken seriously and adequately evaluated. Several of the skills of active listening are valuable in discussing physical, psychological, and social issues with patients. These skills have been clearly shown to be linked to recognition of emotional problems when used by general practitioners.

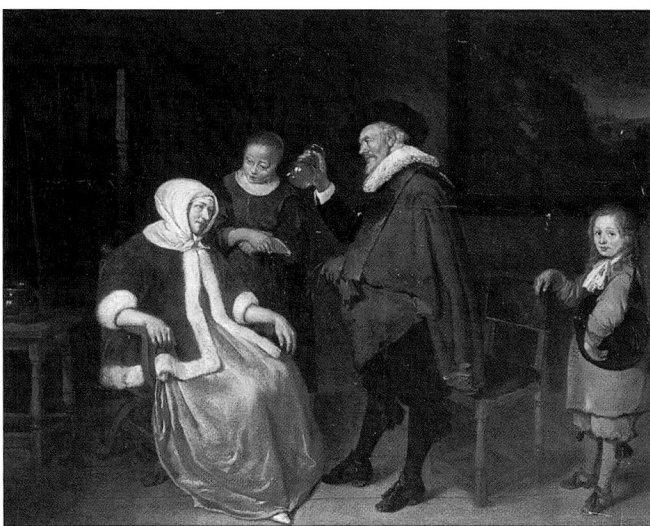

Visiting the sick woman, by Quiringh Gerritsz van Brekelenkam (c 1620-68)

Three functions of the medical consultation

1 Build the relationship
- Greet the patient warmly and by name
- Active listening
- Detect and respond to emotional issues

2 Collect data
- Do not interrupt patient
- Consider other factors
- Elicit patient's explanatory model
- Develop shared understanding

3 Agree a management plan
- Provide information
- Make links
- Appropriate use of reassurance
- Negotiate behaviour change
- Negotiate a management plan

Responding to patients' "cues"

Verbal cues
- State your observation—"You say that recently you have been feeling fed-up and irritable"
- Repeat the patient's own words—"Not well since your mother died"
- Seek clarification—"What do you mean when you say you always feel tired?"

Non-verbal cues
- Comment on your observation—"I can hear tears in your voice"
- Ask a question—"I wonder if that upsets you more than you like to admit?"

Aspects of interview style that aid assessment of patients' emotional problems

Early in the interview
- Make good eye contact
- Clarify presenting complaint
- Use directive questions for physical complaints
- Begin with open ended questions, moving to closed questions later

Interview style
- Make empathic comments
- Pick up verbal cues
- Pick up non-verbal cues
- Do not read notes while taking patient's history
- Deal with over-talkativeness
- Ask more questions about the history of the emotional problem

Active listening skills

Open ended questions—Questions that cannot be answered in one word require patient to expand

Open-to-closed cones—Move towards closed questions at the end of a section of the consultation

Checking—Repeat back to patient to ensure that you have understood

Facilitation—Encourage patient both verbally ("Go on") and non-verbally (nodding)

Legitimising patient's feelings—"This is clearly worrying you a great deal," followed by, "You have an awful lot to cope with," or, "I think most people would feel the same way"

Surveying the field—Repeated signals that further details are wanted: "Is there anything else?"

Empathic comments—"This is clearly worrying you a great deal"

Offering support—"I am worried about you, and I want to know how I can help you best with this problem"

Negotiating priorities—If there are several problems draw up a list and negotiate which to deal with first

Summarising—Check what was reported and use as a link to next part of interview. This helps to develop a shared understanding of the problems and to control flow of interview if there is too much information

Eliciting a patient's explanatory model

When people consult a doctor, they do so with explanatory ideas about their problems and with anxieties and concerns that reflect these ideas. They are also likely to have hopes and expectations concerning the care that they will receive. It is important not to make assumptions about patients' health beliefs, concerns, and expectations but to elicit these as a basis for providing information and negotiating a management plan.

People's health beliefs and behaviours develop and are sustained within families, and families are deeply affected by the illness of a family member. "Thinking family" can help to avoid difficult and frustrating interactions with family members.

Providing information

Doctors should consider three key questions when providing information to a patient:
• What does the patient already know?
• What does the patient want to know?
• What does the patient need to know?

The first question emphasises the importance of building on the patient's existing explanatory model, adding to what he or she already knows, and correcting inaccuracies. The second and third reflect the need to address two agendas, the patient's and the doctor's. In addition, it is important for the doctor to show ongoing concern and emotional support, making empathic comments, legitimising the patient's concerns, and offering support.

Negotiating a management plan

The ideal management plan is one that reflects current best evidence on treatment, is tailored to the situation and preferences of the patient, and addresses emotional and social issues. Both patient and doctor should be involved in developing the plan, although one or the other may have the greater input depending on the nature of the problem and the inclinations of the patient.

Appropriate use of reassurance

Reassurance is effective only when doctors understand exactly what it is that their patients fear and when they address these fears truthfully and accurately. Often it is not possible to reassure patients about the diagnosis or outcome of disease, but it is always possible to provide support and to show personal concern for them.

Dealing with difficult emotions: denial, anger, and fear

Denial—When patients deny the seriousness of their illness you should never be tempted to force them into facing it. The decision on how to address denial must be based on how adaptive the denial is, what kind of support is available to the patient, and how well prepared the patient is to deal with the fears that underlie the denial.

Think family

When interviewing an individual
● Ask how family members view the problem
● Ask about impact of the problem on family function
● Discuss implications of management plan for the family

When a family member comes in with patient
● Acknowledge relative's presence
● Check that patient is comfortable with relative's presence
● Clarify reasons for relative coming
● Ask for relative's observations and opinions of the problem
● Solicit relative's help in treatment if appropriate
● If patient is an adolescent accompanied by an adult always spend part of consultation without the adult present
● Never take sides

Negotiating a management plan

Ascertain expectations
● What does patient know?
● What does patient want?—Investigation? Management? Outcomes?

Advise on options
● Elicit patient's preferences

Develop a plan
● Involve patient
● Tailor preferred option to patient's needs and situation
● "Think family"

Check understanding
● Ensure that patient is clear about plan
● Consider a written summary

Advise on contingency management
● What should patient do if things do not go according to plan?

Agree arrangements for follow up and review

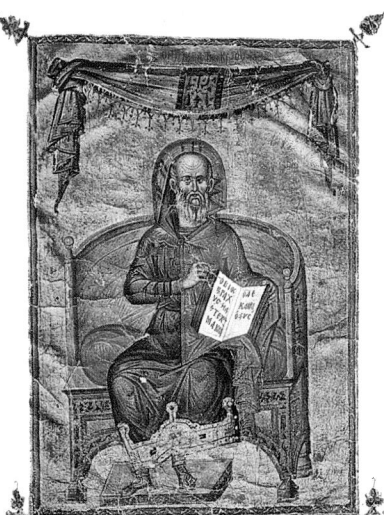

Reassurance is an essential skill of bedside medicine. (Hippocrates (469-399 BC), the "father of bedside medicine")

Anger—If patients or relatives become angry, try to avoid being defensive. Acknowledge the feelings that are expressed and ask about the reasons for these. Take concerns seriously and indicate that you will take appropriate action.

Fear—Many patients are frightened that they may have some serious disease. It is crucial to ensure that you have addressed what a patient is really worried about as well as checking that the patient has correctly understood what you are concerned about.

Motivation

Efforts to help people reduce alcohol consumption, stop smoking, and manage chronic illness have highlighted the importance of good interviewing skills in motivating patients to change their behaviour. This is not to say that patients no longer have the responsibility for such change, but doctors should recognise that they bear some responsibility for ensuring that patients get the best possible help in arriving at the decision to change.

Making the link between emotions and physical symptoms

Particular strategies may be needed to help people who present with physical symptoms of psychological distress but who have not made the link between these and their emotional and life problems. However, it is essential that you do not go faster than the patient and try to force the patient to accept your explanation.

Feeling understood—Ensuring that the patient feels understood is essential. It is crucial to get the patient on your side and show that you are taking his or her problems seriously. Start from the patient's viewpoint and find out what the patient thinks may be causing the symptoms, while at the same time picking up any verbal and non-verbal cues of emotional distress.

Broadening the agenda can begin when all the information has been gathered. The aim is to broaden the agenda from one where the problem is seen essentially as physical to one where both physical and psychological problems can be acknowledged. Acknowledging the reality of the patient's pain or other symptoms is essential and must be done sensitively. Summarise by reminding the patient of all the symptoms, both physical and emotional, that you have elicited and link them to life events if this is possible.

Negotiating explanations can involve various techniques. Only one or two will be appropriate for each patient, and different techniques may be useful at different times. Simple explanation is the commonest, but it is insufficient to say "Anxiety causes headaches." A three stage explanation is required in which anxiety is linked to muscle tension, which then causes pain. A similar approach can be used to explain how depression causes lowering of the pain threshold, which results in pain being felt more severely than it otherwise would be.

Once the patient and doctor have agreed that psychological distress is an important factor in the patient's illness, they can start to examine management options to address this. Even if the patient has significant physical disease, it is important to detect and manage psychological comorbidity.

Visiting the sick woman is held at the Hermitage and is reproduced with permission of Bridgeman Art Library.

Helping patients to change their behaviour

Explore motivation for change
- Build rapport and be neutral
- Help draw up list of problems and priorities
- Is problem behaviour on patient's agenda?
- If not, raise it sensitively
- Does patient consider the behaviour to be a problem?
- Do others?

Clarify patient's view of the problem
- Help draw up a balance sheet of pros and cons
- Empathise with difficulty of changing
- Reinforce statements that express a desire to change
- Resist saying why you think patient ought to change
- Summarise frequently
- Discuss statements that are contradictory

Promote resolution
If no change is wanted negotiate if, when, and how to review
- Enable informed decision making
- Give basic information about safety or risks of behaviour
- Provide results of any examination or test
- Highlight potential medical, legal, or social consequences
- Explain likely outcome of potential choices or interventions
- Get feedback from patient
- Give patient responsibility for decision

Key stages in linking somatic symptoms of emotional distress

- Helping patient to feel understood
- Broadening agenda to cover physical, psychological, and social issues
- Negotiating explanations for how physical symptoms, psychological distress, and social problems may be linked via physiological mechanisms

Evidence based summary

- The style with which a doctor listens to a patient will influence what the patient says
- Effective communication between doctor and patient leads to improved outcome for many common diseases
- Patients' compliance will be improved if the management plan has been negotiated jointly

Lang F, Floyd MR, Beine KL. Clues to patients' explanations and concerns about their illnesses—a call for active listening. *Arch Fam Med* 2000;9:222-7

Stewart MA. Effective physician-patient communication and health outcomes: a review. *Can Med Assoc J* 1995;152:1423-33

Roter D, Hall JA, Merisca R, Nordstron B, Cretin D, Svarstad B. Effectiveness of interventions to improve patient compliance: a meta-analysis. *Med Care* 1998;36:1138-61

Further reading

- Cole SA, Bird J. *The medical interview: the three function approach.* St Louis, MO: Harcourt Health Sciences, 2000
- Gask L, Morriss R, Goldberg D. *Reattribution: managing somatic presentation of emotional distress.* 2nd ed. Manchester: University of Manchester, 2000. (Teaching videotape available from Nick.Jordan@man.ac.uk)
- Usherwood T. *Understanding the consultation.* Milton Keynes: Open University Press, 1999

2 Beginning treatment

Jonathan Price, Laurence Leaver

Traditionally, the management of newly presenting patients has two stages—assessment and then treatment. However, this two stage approach has limitations. When underlying disease pathology is diagnosed there may be delays in starting effective treatment. If no disease is found reassurance is often ineffective. In both cases many patients are left feeling uncertain and dissatisfied. Lack of immediate information and agreed plans may mean that patients and their families become anxious and draw inappropriate conclusions, and an opportunity to engage them fully in their management is missed.

If simple diagnosis is supplemented with fuller explanation, patient satisfaction and outcomes are improved. This can be achieved by integrating assessment and treatment. The aim of an integrated consultation is that the patient leaves with a clear understanding of the likely diagnosis, feeling that concerns have been addressed, and knowledge of the treatment and prognosis (that is, the assessment becomes part of the treatment). This approach can be adopted in primary and secondary care and can be applied to patients with or without an obvious disease explanation for their symptoms. The integrated approach may require more time, but this is offset by a likely reduction in patients' subsequent attendance and use of resources.

This article describes principles and practical procedures for effective communication and simple interventions. They can be applied to various clinical situations—such as straightforward single consultation, augmenting brief medical care, and promoting an effective start to continuing treatment and care.

General principles

Integrating physical and psychological care
Somatic symptoms are subjective and have two components, a somatic element (a bodily sensation due to physiology or pathology) and a psychological element (related to thoughts and beliefs about the symptoms). Traditional management focuses only on the somatic component, with the aim of detecting and treating underlying pathology. Addressing the psychological component in the consultation as well, with simple psychological interventions, is likely to reduce distress and disability and reduce the need for subsequent specialist treatment.

Providing continuity
Seeing the same doctor on each visit increases patient satisfaction. Continuity may also improve medical outcomes, including distress, compliance, preventive care, and resource use. Problems resulting from lack of continuity can be minimised by effective communication between doctors.

Involving the patient
The psychological factors of beliefs and attitudes about illness and treatment are major determinants of outcome. Hence, strategies that increase understanding, sense of control, and participation in treatment can have large benefits. One example is written management plans agreed between doctor and patient. This approach is the basis of the Department of Health's "Expert Patient Programme," which aims to help patients to "act as experts in managing their own condition, with appropriate support from health and social care services."

Mismatch of expectations and experiences

What patients want	What some patients get
To know the cause	No diagnosis
Explanation and information	Poor explanation that does not address their needs and concerns
Advice and treatment	Inadequate advice
Reassurance	Lack of reassurance
To be taken seriously by a sympathetic and competent doctor	Feeling that doctor is uninterested or believes symptoms are unimportant

---

Disease centred versus patient centred consultations

Disease centred—Doctor concentrates on standard medical agenda of diagnosis through systematic inquiries about patient's symptoms and medical history

Patient centred—Doctor works to patient's agenda, including listening and allowing patient to explain all the reasons for attending, feelings, and expectations. Decision making may be shared, and plans are explicit and agreed. Patient centred consultations need take no longer than traditional disease centred consultations

---

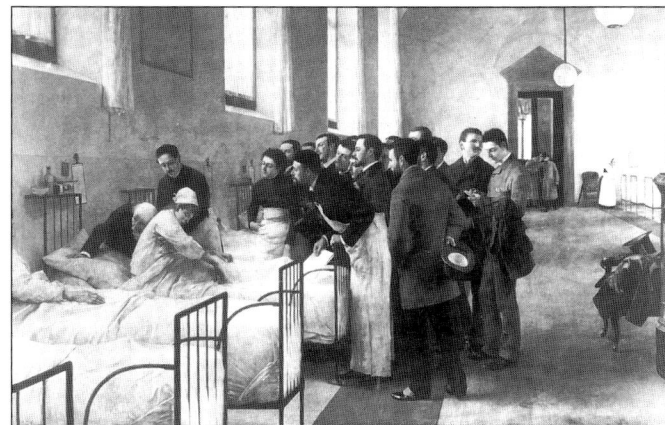

Taking time to listen to and address patients' ideas, concerns, and expectations can improve outcomes (*Charcot at the Saltpêtrière* by Luis Jimenez y Aranda, 1889, in the Provincial Museum of Art, Seville)

Communication between doctors

- Reduce need for communication between doctors by providing continuity of care whenever possible
- Brief, structured letters are more likely to be read than lengthy, unstructured letters
- Letters from primary to secondary care should provide relevant background information and a clear reason for referral
- Letters from secondary to primary care should provide only essential information, address the needs of referrer, and outline a proposed management plan and what has been discussed with patient
- Avoid using letters for medical records purposes rather than communication
- The telephone can be a prompt and effective means of communication and is particularly useful in complex cases

Thinking "family"

Relatives' illness beliefs and attitudes are also crucial to outcome and are therefore worth addressing. Key people may be invited to join a consultation (with the patient's permission) and their concerns identified, acknowledged, and addressed. Actively involving relatives, who will spend more time with the patient than will the doctor, allows them to function as co-therapists.

Effective communication

Gaining and demonstrating understanding

Simple techniques can be used to improve communication. The first two stages of the three function approach (see previous article) are appropriate. The first stage is building a relationship in which a patient gives his or her history and feels understood. The second stage is for the doctor to share his or her understanding of the illness with the patient. In cases that are more complicated it may be most effective to add an additional brief session with a practice or clinic nurse.

Providing information for patients

Patients require information about the likely cause of their illness, details of any test results and their meaning, and a discussion of possible treatments. Even when this information has been given in a consultation, however, many patients do not understand or remember what they are told. Hence, the provision of simple written information can be a time efficient way of improving patient outcomes.

One way of providing written information is to copy correspondence such as referral and assessment letters to the patient concerned. For those not used to doing this, it may seem a challenge, but any changes needed to make the letters understandable (and acceptable) to patients are arguably desirable in any case. Letters should be clearly structured, medical jargon minimised, pejorative terms omitted, and common words that may be misinterpreted (such as "chronic") explained.

Well written patient information materials (leaflets and books) are available, as are guidelines for their development. The National Electronic Library of Health (www.nelh.nhs.uk) is a new internet resource that aims to provide high quality information for healthcare consumers and is linked to NHS Direct Online (www.nhsdirect.nhs.uk/main.jhtml). There are also many books to recommend—such as *Chronic Fatigue Syndrome (CFS/ME): The Facts* (see Further reading list). Information is most helpful if it addresses not only the nature of the problem, its prognosis, and treatment options, but also self care and ways of coping.

The assessment as treatment

Reassurance

Worry about health (health anxiety) is a common cause of distress and disability in those with and without serious disease. Reassurance is therefore a key component of starting treatment.

The first step is to elicit and acknowledge patients' expectations, concerns, and illness beliefs. This is followed by history taking, examination, and if necessary investigation. Premature reassurance (such as "I'm sure its nothing much") may be construed as the doctor not taking the problem seriously. Finally, the explanation should address all of a patient's concerns and is best based on the patient's understanding of how his or her body functions, which may differ from the doctor's.

A modest increase in consultation time, provision of written information, and perhaps the use of trained nursing staff to

---

Gaining understanding of patients' concerns

- Read referral letter or notes, or both, before seeing patient
- Encourage patients to discuss their presenting concerns without interruption or premature closure
- Explore patients' presenting complaints, concerns, and understanding (beliefs)
- Inquire about disability
- Inquire about self care activities
- Show support and empathy
- Use silence appropriately
- Use non-verbal communication such as eye contact, nods, and leaning forward

---

Showing your understanding of patients' concerns

- Relay key messages—such as, "The symptoms are real," "We will look after you," and "You're not alone"
- Take patients seriously and make sure they know it
- Don't dismiss presenting complaints, whether or not relevant pathology is found
- Explain your understanding of the problem—what it is, what it isn't, treatment, and the future. A diagram may help
- Consider offering a positive explanation in the absence of relevant physical pathology
- Reassure
- Avoid mixed messages
- Encourage and answer questions
- Share decisions
- Communicate the management plan effectively, both verbally and in writing
- Provide self care information, including advice on lifestyle change
- Explain how to get routine or emergency follow up, and what to look out for that would change the management plan

---

Providing information

- Invite and answer questions
- Use lay terms, and build on patient's understanding of illness wherever possible
- Avoid medical jargon and terms with multiple meanings, such as "chronic"
- Involve relatives
- Provide written material when available
- Provide a written management plan when appropriate

The complexity of reassurance

General reassurance
- To know it will be OK
- To know I will be looked after
- To know there are others like me

Reassurance about cause
- To know what it is
- To know what it is not
- To know it's not serious
  "There are several possible causes, not just cancer"
  "It's not cancer"
  "It will get better"

Reassurance about cure
- To know it can be treated
- To know it will be treated
- To know how it will be treated
- To know the complaint will go away

facilitate information giving, can all enhance doctor-patient communication and, therefore, reassurance. Although extra time and effort may be needed, it may well reduce subsequent demand on resources.

Being positive

Doctors themselves are potentially powerful therapeutic agents. There is evidence that being deliberately positive in a consultation may increase this effect. In one randomised trial, general practice patients received either a positive consultation (firm diagnosis and good prognosis) or a non-positive consultation (no firm diagnosis and uncertain prognosis). Two weeks later, the positive consultation, which was simple and brief, had improved symptoms, with a number needed to treat of four (95% confidence interval 3 to 9).

Using tests as treatment

Tests should ideally be informative and reassuring for both doctors and patients. However, there is increasing evidence that tests may not reassure some patients and may even increase their anxiety. This is most likely with patients who are already anxious about their health. When weighing the pros and cons of ordering a test, doctors should take account of the potential psychological impact on their patient (both positive and negative).

Providing explanations after negative investigation

Even when tests are reported as normal, some patients are not reassured. Such patients may benefit from an explanation of what is wrong with them, not just what is not wrong. A cognitive behavioural model can be used to explain how interactions between physiology, thoughts, and emotion can cause symptoms without pathology. Simple headache provides an analogy: the pain is real, and often distressing and disabling, but is usually associated with "stress." Diagnoses such as "tension headache" and "irritable bowel syndrome" can be helpful in reducing patients' anxiety about sinister causes for their symptoms.

Planning for the future

Maintaining and increasing activities

Sometimes patients unnecessarily avoid or reduce their activities for fear it will make their illness worse. This coping strategy magnifies disability. Planning a graded return towards normal activities is one of the most effective ways of helping such patients. A plan should specify clearly what activity, for how long, when, with whom, and how often. It is best if the plan is written down and reviewed regularly. A collaborative approach increases the chances of success.

Follow up

Positively following up patients who have presented for the first time can be an effective use of time. It allows review and modification of the management plan and may be particularly effective if the same doctor is seen.

The painting of Charcot is reproduced with permission of the Wellcome Library.

Characteristics of brief psychological intervention

- Brief, single session intervention
- Suitable for more complex problems, such as in secondary care
- Delivered with or soon after clinic attendance
- Integrated with usual care
- Uses cognitive understanding of health anxiety
- Minimises negative aspects of patient experience
- Reinforces positive aspects of patient experience
- Provides explicit explanation and reassurance

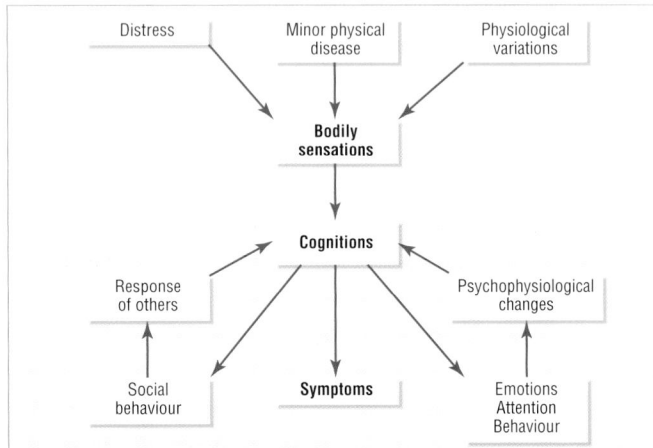

A simple cognitive model of physical symptoms. A cognitive model is one in which the patient's thoughts and beliefs are seen as central to the aetiology, perception, and presentation of the problem

Evidence based summary

- The quality of communication, both in history taking and in discussing a management plan, influences patient outcome
- Patients should be encouraged to take an active role in maintaining or improving their own health, and doctors should ensure they are given the necessary information and opportunities for self management
- Reassurance involves eliciting and acknowledging patients' expectations, concerns, and illness beliefs

Coulter A, Entwistle V, Gilbert D. Sharing decisions with patients: is the information good enough? *BMJ* 1999;318:318-22

Di Blasi Z, Harkness E, Ernst E, Georgiou A, Kleijnen J. Influence of context effects on health outcomes: a systematic review. *Lancet* 2001;357:575-762

Stewart M. Effective physician-patient communication and health outcomes: a review. *Can Med Assoc J* 1995;152:1423-33

Thomas KB. General practice consultations: is there any point in being positive? *BMJ* 1997;294:1200-2

Further reading

- Balint M. *The doctor, his patient, and the illness.* Tunbridge Wells: Pitman Medical, 1957
- Department of Health. *The NHS plan—A plan for investment. A plan for reform.* London: DoH, 2000
- Campling F, Sharpe M. *Chronic fatigue syndrome (CFS/ME): the facts.* Oxford: Oxford University Press, 2000
- Department of Health. *The expert patient: a new approach to chronic disease management for the 21st century.* 2001 (www.ohn.gov.uk/ohn/people/ep_report.pdf

3 Organising care for chronic illness

Michael Von Korff, Russell E Glasgow, Michael Sharpe

A major and increasing task for health services is the management of chronic illness. Although the details of chronic illness management will depend on the illness in question, many of the principles are common to all chronic conditions.

Principles of effective management

Whatever health services may offer, most of the day to day responsibilities for the care of chronic illness fall on patients and their families. Planners and organisers of medical care must therefore recognise that health care will be most effective if it is delivered in collaboration with patients and their families. To enable patients to play an active role in their care, health services must not only provide good medical treatment but also improve patients' knowledge and self management skills. This can be done by supplementing medical care with educational and cognitive behavioural interventions. Chronic disease treatment programmes have tended to underestimate the need for this aspect of care, and, consequently, many treatment programmes have been psychologically naive and, as a result, less effective than they could have been.

Services also need to be not merely reactive to patients' requests but proactive with planned follow up. Finally, to be most efficient, interventions are best organised in a stepped fashion—that is, the more complex and expensive interventions are given only when simpler and cheaper ones have been shown to be inadequate or inappropriate.

Collaboration with patients and families

To win the collaboration of patients and their families, those providing care need to elicit, negotiate and agree on a definition of the problem they are working on with each patient. They must then agree on the targets and goals for management and develop an individualised collaborative self management plan. This plan should be based on established cognitive behavioural principles and on the evidence relating to the management of the chronic condition.

In order to implement collaborative care, patients and their families require access to the necessary information and services to enable them to play a full and informed role. The need for collaborative care in which patients play an active role has been highlighted in Britain with the development of the concept of the "expert patient."

Encouraging self care

Active self care is critical to the optimal management of chronic illness. Interventions to optimise self care are based on cognitive behavioural principles.

They start with an assessment of patients' attitudes and beliefs about their illness and their chosen coping behaviours. This assessment then guides the provision of information, the resolution of misunderstandings and misinterpretations, and collaborative goal setting. These are agreed between patient and members of the healthcare team.

The outcome of this initial assessment takes the form of a personal action plan, a written agreement between those delivering care and the patient. The patient keeps a copy of the plan, and the healthcare team keeps another. The plan can be written on brief, standardised forms. The plan is not static but is

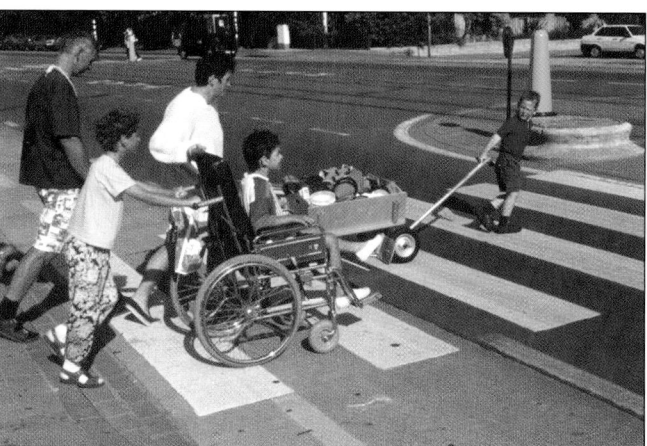
Treating chronic conditions must involve the family

Common elements of effective chronic illness management

- Collaboration between service providers and patients
- A personalised written care plan
- Tailored education in self management
- Planned follow up
- Monitoring of outcome and adherence to treatment
- Targeted use of specialist consultation of referral
- Protocols for stepped care

Principles of collaboration

- Understanding of patients' beliefs, wishes, and circumstances
- Understanding of family beliefs and needs
- Identification of a single person to be main link with each patient
- Collaborative definition of problems and goals
- Negotiated agreed plans regularly reviewed
- Active follow up with patients
- Regular team review

The UK "expert patient" programme*

- Encouragement of self care protocols, nationally and locally
- Development of electronic and written self care material
- Training programmes, national and local
- Integrating self care into local health planning
- Nurse led telephone service (NHS Direct)

* From: Department of Health. *The expert patient: a new approach to chronic disease management for the 21st century* (www.ohn.gov.uk/ohn/people/expert)

developed over time: the initial goals and the care plan designed to achieve them are refined in view of the patient's progress and the identification of factors that are either helpful or unhelpful in achieving the desired outcome.

Active follow up
The personal action plan guides the patient's follow up contacts. Active planned follow up ensures that the plan is carried out and that modifications to it are made as needed. These steps are repeated in an iterative, ongoing, and flexible way rather than all at once in a single visit. Because the care of chronic illness is a long term process, the work of supporting self care does not need to be done all at once but can be spread over many contacts.

Individualised stepped care
Stepped care provides a framework for using limited resources to greatest effect. Professional care is stepped in intensity—that is, it starts with limited professional input and systematic monitoring and is then augmented for patients who do not achieve an acceptable outcome. Initial and subsequent treatments are selected according to evidence based guidelines in light of a patient's progress.

The principle of increasing intensity of professional input for those who do not respond to initial management is familiar in primary care. However, organised stepped care requires the systematic monitoring of progress and higher levels of coordination between specialist care, care management, and primary care than generally exist. The primary care team, a specialist consultant (when needed), and a care manager (when needed) work together to provide the level of professional support needed to achieve a favourable outcome. Stepped care is individualised according to each patient's preferences and progress.

Skills required by those delivering care

The team providing care must not only be familiar with a patient's condition but must also possess the psychological skills to help the patient achieve self care. They also need access to specialists in psychological and psychiatric management to provide supervision and consultation in selected cases. The necessary psychological skills include
- Anxiety management
- Recognition and treatment of depression
- Cognitive behavioural analysis
- Cognitive behavioural principles of step by step change
- Ability to monitor patient's progress.

Changes in the organisation of care

Achieving collaboration between healthcare providers and chronically ill patients requires organisational changes in six related areas.

Organisation of care—Clinical leadership should encourage efforts to improve quality, including development of incentives for improved care and reorganisation of acute care to encourage self care.

Clinical information systems—A disease (or disorder) registry should be set up that identifies the population to be served and includes information on the performance of guideline based care, including self care tasks. The registry should permit identification of patients with specific needs, reminder systems, and tailored treatment planning.

Plan for collaborative self care

1 **Assessment**
- Assess patient's self management beliefs, attitudes, and knowledge
- Identify personal barriers and supports
- Collaborate in setting goals
- Develop individually tailored strategies and problem solving

2 **Goal setting and personal action plan**
- List goals in behavioural terms
- Identify barriers to implementation
- Make plans that address barriers to progress
- Provide a follow up plan
- Share the plan with all members of the healthcare team

3 **Active follow up to monitor progress and support patient**

Levels of stepped care

1 Systematic routine assessment and preventive maintenance
2 Self care with low intensity support
3 Care management in primary care
4 Intensive care management with specialist advice
5 Specialist care

Assumptions of stepped care

- Different individuals require different levels of care
- The optimal level of care is determined by monitoring outcomes
- Moving from lower to higher levels of care based on patient outcomes can increases effectiveness and lower costs

---

Example of changes in organisation of care for patients with diabetes

Organisation of care
- Primary care clinic initiates year long effort to reorganise diabetes care
- Team is set up and meets regularly to make changes, monitor progress, and address obstacles

Clinical information systems
- Team develops a register of all patients with diabetes in the clinic, with records of HbA_{1C} values, eye and foot examinations, and goals and key elements of patients' personal action plans

Delivery system design
- Clinic nurses assigned responsibility for diabetes case management
- Doctors agree to provide planned visits for all diabetic patients at least once a year, including preventive services (such as eye and foot examinations, ordering HbA_{1C} tests, screening for depression)
- Clinic support staff maintain the register and print out a status report before each visit

Decision support
- Team agrees on standard evidence based guidelines and adapts them to clinic and liaison with the specialist diabetic clinic
- Team agrees a standard form for planned visits

Community resources
- Nurse case managers plan training in diabetes self management. The nurses are trained to co-lead the course at regular intervals

Self care support
- Nurse case managers decide that every diabetic patient will have a personal action plan developed within a year
- Each nurse sees one patient a week until this goal is accomplished
- Nurses telephone patients who have not been seen for six months and those who need extra support to achieve their goals

Delivery system design—Practice team roles should be changed in the organisation of visits and in follow up care. Useful innovations include group visits, planned visits, and telephone delivered care.

Decision support—Evidence based practice guidelines and protocols should be made effective by integrating information and reminders into visits. There should be collaborative support from relevant medical specialties.

Community resources—Links should be established with community resources, especially for vulnerable populations such as elderly, low income, and deprived populations.

Self care support—Tailored educational resources, skills training, and psychosocial support are effective. Successful self care programmes rely on collaboration; patient centred interventions for managing illness are especially beneficial.

Is this approach feasible for the large numbers of patients seen in busy primary and secondary care settings? There is growing experience with integrating support for self care to the delivery of routine medical care. Specific techniques such as cognitive behavioural interventions and the use of nurses and other staff as care managers have been found to be both feasible and effective. However, the full implementation of this approach in primary care requires substantial organisational changes. These enable medical and other expertise to be used more effectively and efficiently. They also enable doctors to obtain greater satisfaction in being responsible for higher quality care.

Evidence that it works

Collaborative self care has been used to guide efforts to improve the quality of chronic illness care in many different healthcare settings and for many different chronic conditions including diabetes, heart failure, geriatric care, depression, and asthma. This approach gives patients the confidence and skills for self care and for getting what they need from the healthcare system (that is, becoming active, informed patients). Such effective support of patients is more likely to occur when the providers of care themselves have the information, training, resources, and time to deliver effective interventions (that is, are a well prepared, proactive practice team).

There is now considerable evidence and practical experience that supports fundamental changes in the way we organise and deliver health care to better support patients who are living with a chronic condition. Consequently, we need to include psychological and behavioural expertise as essential supplements to basic medical treatment.

Patient centred care is more than a respectful attitude or a style of clinical interviewing. It means that healthcare systems are organised to maximise the effectiveness of patients to manage their chronic illness themselves.

Psychological medicine will make its full contribution only when an awareness of the importance of psychological and behavioural factors is fully integrated into general medical care.

Work on this article was supported by grants from the Robert Wood Johnson Foundation National Program for Improving Chronic Illness Care, NIMH grants MH51338 and MH41739, and NIH grant P01 DE08773.

The picture is reproduced with permission of CC Studio/SPL.

Making evidence based care time and cost effective

Problems
- Time for patient care
- Time for assessing evidence
- Unrealistic patient expectations and demands
- Lack of patient understanding of behavioural basis of self care
- Lack of involvement of patients in clinical decisions
- Lack of professional skills
- Access to disparate community and medical services

Solutions
- Treatment protocols
- Involvement of healthcare team
- Use of self help procedures
- Formalising links with local health, social, and voluntary agencies
- Liaison with specialist medical, psychiatric, and psychological services
- Continuing professional development

Evidence based summary
- Collaborative and adaptive approaches to self care that are structured and integrated into medical services improve outcomes for many chronic diseases
- Systematic setting of therapeutic goals and monitoring of clinical treatment and outcomes are integral to this approach
- Such an approach to health care will often require changes to the way in which teams and primary and secondary care services interact

Department of Health. *The expert patient: a new approach to chronic disease management for the 21st century* (www.ohn.gov.uk/ohn/people/ep_report.pdf)

Gibson PG, Coughlan J, Wilson AJ, Abramson M, Bauman A, Hensley MJ, et al. Self-management education and regular practitioner review for adults with asthma. *Cochrane Database Syst Rev* 2000;(2): CD001117

Further reading
- Department of Health. *The expert patient: a new approach to chronic disease management for the 21st century.* (www.ohn.gov.uk/ohn/people/ep_report.pdf)
- Lorig KR, Sobel DS, Stewart AL, Brown BW Jr, Bandura A, Ritter P, et al. Evidence suggesting that a chronic disease self-management program can improve health status while reducing hospitalisation. *Med Care* 1999;37:5-14
- Von Korff M, Gruman J, Schaefer J, Curry S, Wagner EH. Collaborative management of chronic illness. *Ann Intern Med* 1997; 127:1097-102
- Wagner EH, Glasgow RE, Davis C, Bonomi AE, Provost L, McCulloch D, et al. Quality improvement in chronic illness care: a collaborative approach. *Jt Comm J Qual Improv* 2001;27:63-80
- Wolpert HA, Anderson BJ. Management of diabetes: are doctors framing the benefits from the wrong perspective? *BMJ* 2001;323: 994-6

4 Depression in medical patients

Robert Peveler, Alan Carson, Gary Rodin

Depressive illness is usually treatable. It is common and results in marked disability, diminished survival, and increased healthcare costs. As a result, it is essential that all doctors have a basic understanding of its diagnosis and management. In patients with physical illness depression may
- Be a coincidental association
- Be a complication of physical illness
- Cause or exacerbate somatic symptoms (such as fatigue, malaise, or pain).

Clinical features and classification

The term depression describes a spectrum of mood disturbance ranging from mild to severe and from transient to persistent. Depressive symptoms are continuously distributed in any population but are judged to be of clinical significance when they interfere with normal activities and persist for at least two weeks, in which case a diagnosis of a depressive illness or disorder may be made. The diagnosis depends on the presence of two cardinal symptoms of persistent and pervasive low mood and loss of interest or pleasure in usual activities.

Adjustment disorders are milder or more short lived episodes of depression and are thought to result from stressful experiences.

Major depressive disorder refers to a syndrome that requires the presence of five or more symptoms of depression in the same two week period.

Dysthymia covers persistent symptoms of depression that may not be severe enough to meet the criteria for major depression, in which depressed mood is present for two or more years. Such chronic forms of depression are associated with an increased risk of subsequent major depression, considerable social disability, and unhealthy lifestyle choices such as poor diet or cigarette smoking.

Manic depressive (bipolar) disorder relates to the occurrence of episodes of both major depression and mania.

Epidemiology

The World Health Organization estimates that depression will become the second most important cause of disability worldwide (after ischaemic heart disease) by 2020. Major depressive disorder affects 1 in 20 people during their lifetime. Both major depression and dysthymia seem to be more common in women.

Depressive illness is strongly associated with physical disease. Up to a third of physically ill patients attending hospital have depressive symptoms. Depression is even more common in patients with
- Life threatening or chronic physical illness
- Unpleasant and demanding treatment
- Low social support and other adverse social circumstances
- Personal or family history of depression or other psychological vulnerability
- Alcoholism and substance misuse
- Drug treatments that cause depression as a side effect, such as antihypertensives, corticosteroids, and chemotherapy agents.

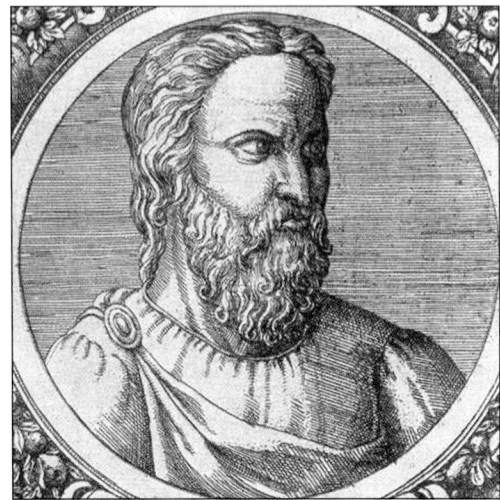

Aretaeus of Cappadocia (circa 81-138 AD) is credited with the first clinical description of depression

Criteria for major depression*

Five or more of the following symptoms during the same two week period representing a change from normal
- Depressed mood†
- Substantial weight loss or weight gain
- Insomnia or hypersomnia
- Feelings of worthlessness or inappropriate guilt
- Recurrent thoughts of death or suicide or suicide attempt
- Decreased interest or pleasure†
- Psychomotor retardation or agitation
- Fatigue or loss of energy
- Diminished ability to think or concentrate

*From *Diagnostic and Statistical Manual of Mental Disorders*, fourth edition
†One of these symptoms must be present

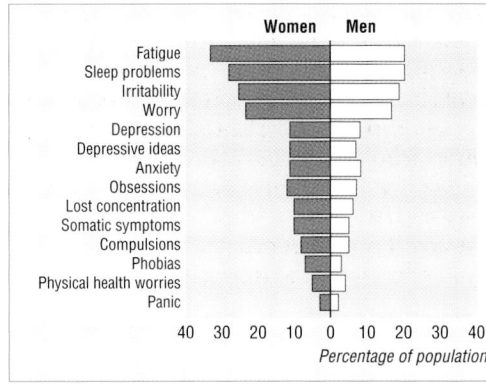

"Neurotic" symptoms, including depression, are continuously distributed in the UK population

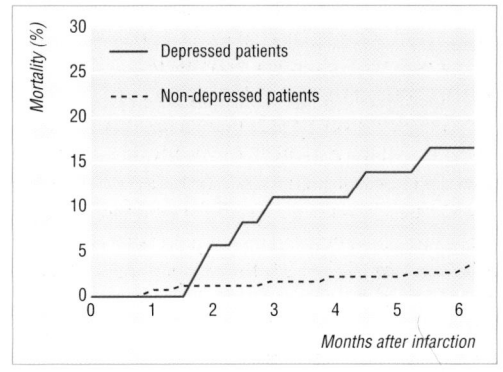

The association between depression and mortality after myocardial infarction

Risk factors

Anxiety, sadness, and somatic discomfort are part of the normal psychological response to life stress, including medical illness. Clinical depression is a final common pathway resulting from the interaction of biological, psychological, and social factors. The likelihood of this outcome depends on such factors as genetic and family predisposition, the clinical course of a concurrent medical illness, the nature of the treatment, functional disability, the effectiveness of individual coping strategies, and the availability of social and other support.

In the attempts to understand the relation between physical illness and depression there has been much debate about the direction of causality. In particular, there has been speculation that certain illnesses—such as stroke, Parkinson's disease, multiple sclerosis, and pancreatic cancer—may cause depression via direct biological mechanisms. Stroke has perhaps received the most attention, but studies have failed to convincingly show direct aetiological mechanisms.

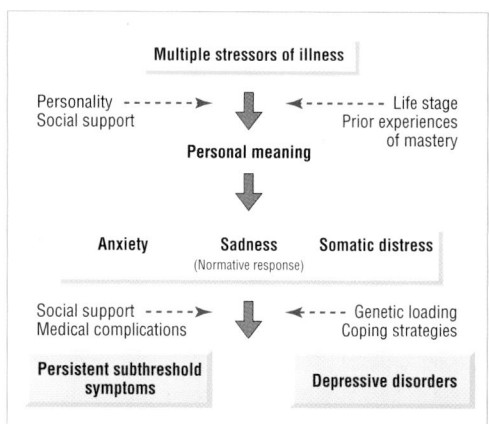

Pathways to depression

Recognition and diagnosis

In spite of its enormous clinical and public health importance, depressive illness is often underdiagnosed and undertreated, particularly when it coexists with physical illness. This often causes great distress for patients who have mistakenly assumed that symptoms such as weakness or fatigue are due to an underlying medical condition.

All medical practitioners must be able to diagnose and manage depressive illness effectively. This depends on
● Alertness to clues in interviews
● Patients' manner
● The use of screening questions in those at risk—in particular, two questions about low mood and lack of pleasure in life can detect up to 95% of patients with major depression.

Self report screening instruments, such as the Beck depression inventory (BDI) and the hospital anxiety and depression scale (HADS) cannot replace systematic clinical assessment, but they are useful in drawing attention to depression and other emotional disturbances in clinical settings where mood is not routinely assessed. Doctors must be aware that persistent low mood and lack of interest and pleasure in life cannot be accounted for by severe physical illness alone. The usual response to illness and treatment is impressive resilience.

If there is doubt about the diagnosis, a doctor may resort to an empirical trial of treatment to establish whether there is benefit. The wider availability of safer drugs and psychological treatments makes this option more attractive than in the past.

Reasons why depression is missed
● Difficulty distinguishing psychological symptoms of depression, such as sadness and loss of interest, from a "realistic" response to stressful physical illness
● Confusion over whether physical symptoms of depression are due to an underlying medical condition
● Negative attitudes to diagnosis of depression
● Unsuitability of clinical setting for discussion of personal and emotional matters
● Patients' unwillingness to report symptoms of depression

Screening questions for depression
● How have you been feeling recently?
● Have you been low in spirits?
● Have you been able to enjoy the things you usually enjoy?
● Have you had your usual level of energy, or have you been feeling tired?
● How has your sleep been?
● Have you been able to concentrate on newspaper articles or your favourite television or radio programmes?

Management

The main aims of treatment are to improve mood and quality of life, reduce the risk of medical complications, improve compliance with and outcome of physical treatment, and facilitate the "appropriate" use of healthcare resources. The development of a treatment plan depends on systematic assessment that should, whenever possible, not only involve the patients but also their partners or other key family members.

Milder or briefer adjustment disorders can be managed by primary care staff without recourse to specialist referral. Education, advice, and reassurance are of value. It is important that primary care staff are familiar with the properties and use of the commoner antidepressant drugs, and the value of brief psychological treatments such as cognitive behaviour therapy, interpersonal therapy, and problem solving.

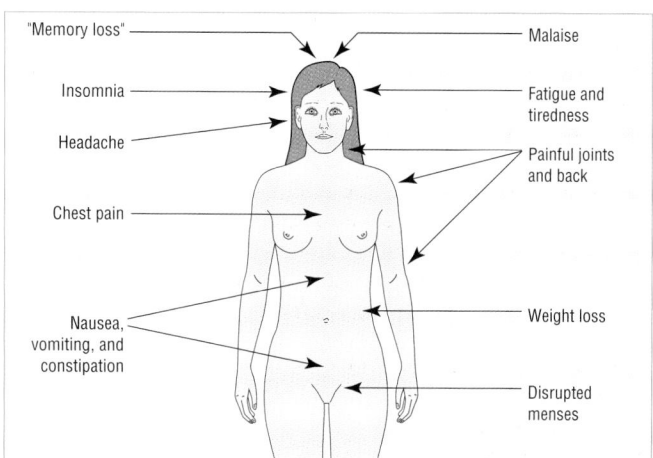

Physical symptoms that may be due to depression

Patients with more enduring or severe symptoms will usually require specific forms of treatment, usually drug treatment. Staff should also be able to assess suicidal thinking and risk. For patients with suicidal ideation or those whose depression has not responded to initial management, specialist referral is the next step in management.

Drug treatment

Antidepressants have been shown to be effective in treating major depressive disorder irrespective of whether the mood disturbance is "understandable." There have been far fewer trials of antidepressants in patients who are also physically unwell, but the available evidence is in keeping with the treatment of depression generally.

One of the commonest questions is which antidepressant should be used. For non-specialists, the range of available drugs, and the claims made about them can be bewildering. There are four main classes of antidepressant
- Tricyclics
- Selective serotonin reuptake inhibitors
- Monoamine oxidase inhibitors
- Others (noradrenaline reuptake inhibitors).

Choice of agent

Data from the Cochrane Collaboration and other systematic reviews show that the differences in overall tolerability between different preparations is minimal. In general, patients are slightly less likely to drop out of trials because of unacceptable side effects when taking a selective serotonin reuptake inhibitor but are slightly less likely to drop out because of treatment inefficacy when taking a tricyclic. Rather than continuously experimenting with a range of different drugs, clinicians should stick to prescribing one drug from each class in order to become familiar with their dosing regimens, actions, interactions, and side effects. Clinicians should also be aware that in certain situations one class of drug may be more advisable than others.

Adequacy of treatment

The debate about different preparations has obscured a potentially more important issue—that of drug dose and compliance. Most prescriptions for antidepressants are for inadequate doses and for inadequate time periods. This problem is compounded by only a minority of patients complying with the prescribed treatment. A recent household survey by the Royal College of Psychiatrists showed that many people believed that antidepressants were addictive and could permanently damage the brain.

Explanation

To treat patients successfully with antidepressants, doctors must be able to show their patient that they have understood the patient's problems, considered the issues, and are advising the best available treatment (see previous chapters). Before starting treatment, patients should be given an explanation of side effects and be reassured that side effects tend to be worse during the first two weeks of treatment and then diminish. They need to be warned that they are unlikely to feel benefits from treatment in the first four weeks. They should be given follow up appointments during this period in order to encourage compliance.

Duration of treatment

After initial treatment has led to remission of symptoms, subsequent treatment can be divided into two phases. Firstly, four to six months of continuous treatment at full dose are

Clinical assessment of suicidal intent

Low level risk

Clinical picture
- Suicidal ideation but no suicide attempts
- Supportive environment
- Physically healthy
- No history of psychiatric illness

Action
Consider referral to mental health professional for routine appointment (not always necessary)

Moderate level risk

Clinical picture
- Low lethality suicide attempt (patient's perception of lethality)
- Frequent thoughts of suicide
- Previous suicide attempts
- Persistent depressive symptoms
- Serious medical illness
- Inadequate social support
- History of psychiatric illness

Action
Refer to mental health professional, to be seen as soon as possible

High level risk

Clinical picture
- Definite plan for suicide (When? Where? How?)
- Major depressive disorder, severe
- High lethality suicide attempt or multiple attempts
- Advanced medical disease
- Social isolation
- History of psychiatric illness

Action
Refer to mental health professional for immediate assessment

Comparison: Antidepressants *v* Placebo
Outcome: Lack of improvement at end of study

Condition	No of patients Drug	No of patients Control	Odds ratio (95% CI)	Weighting (%)	Odds ratio (95% CI)
Cancer	8/36	19/37		11.2	0.29 (0.11 to 0.75)
Cancer	9/28	17/27		9.0	0.30 (0.10 to 0.85)
Diabetes	10/18	12/17		5.4	0.54 (0.14 to 2.07)
Head injury	3/6	3/4		1.7	0.39 (0.03 to 4.54)
Heart disease	1/16	6/8		3.0	0.04 (0.01 to 0.26)
HIV or AIDS	36/50	21/25		8.0	0.52 (0.17 to 1.60)
HIV	22/50	36/47		15.2	0.26 (0.12 to 0.59)
HIV	9/25	11/22		7.6	0.57 (0.18 to 1.80)
Lung disease	8/18	16/18		5.3	0.14 (0.04 to 0.56)
Multiple sclerosis	7/18	8/14		5.2	0.49 (0.12 to 1.95)
Physical illness, elderly	25/39	35/43		10.5	0.42 (0.16 to 1.11)
Physical illness	22/29	21/30		7.7	1.34 (0.43 to 4.18)
Stroke	17/33	24/33		10.2	0.41 (0.15 to 1.10)
Total	177/366	229/325		100.0	0.37 (0.27 to 0.51)

0.1   1   10

Meta-analysis of randomised controlled trials of drug treatment of depression in the physically ill

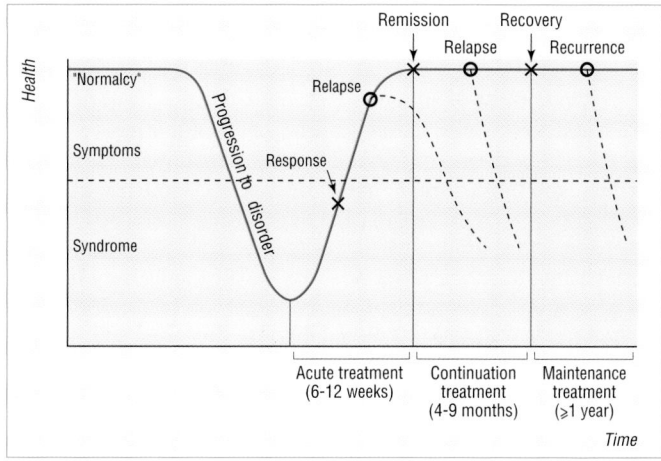

Chart of clinical course indicating remission, recovery, and relapse

necessary to consolidate remission and prevent early relapse. Secondly, consideration must be given to preventive maintenance treatment, to reduce the risks of recurrence of depression. This is usually indicated if the patient has had two or more episodes of depression within the past five years. Psychological treatment may also help to prevent recurrence and can be used in combination with drug treatment.

Psychological treatment

Psychological treatment can range from discussion and simple problem solving to more specialised cognitive or dynamic behavioural psychotherapies. In many cases, brief treatment by non-specialists in primary and secondary care can be effective. Such interventions may include education and reassurance about the common reactions to the threats and losses associated with illness and empathic listening to patients' views, uncertainties, and beliefs about the illness. Education and advice about the medical condition and associated depression may prevent needless worry, reduce feelings of helplessness, and diminish irrational fears. Therapeutic approaches that support or promote active coping strategies are an important aspect of treatment in physically ill patients.

Cognitive behavioural principles may be used by non-specialists to correct distorted thinking and to encourage behaviours that contribute to patients' sense of mastery and wellbeing. Training in briefer forms of treatment using cognitive behavioural principles for primary care staff may be a worthwhile investment.

Cognitive behaviour therapy, interpersonal therapy, and problem solving have all been shown to be effective for treating depression, although there has been only limited evaluation of their effectiveness in physically ill populations. Although time consuming by comparison with drug treatment, psychological treatment may reduce relapse rates and may be cost effective in the long run. Some patients may require preliminary treatment with drugs to enable them to make best use of psychological treatment.

Service organisation

Depression is so common in physically ill patients that it is not feasible for all cases to be managed by mental health specialists. There are advantages to collaborative management with primary care staff working closely with mental health specialists. Community based mental health services may be less accessible to general hospitals and often lack specialist knowledge about assessment and treatment when an important physical illness is also present. Liaison psychiatry services are often well placed to provide support, training, and psychiatric expertise to general hospital patients in a timely fashion.

Problem solving in psychological treatment

- Define and list the problems
- Choose a problem for action
- List alternative courses of action
- Evaluate courses of action and choose the best
- Try the action
- Evaluate the results
- Repeat until major problems have been solved

Evidence based summary

- Depressive illness is an important cause of morbidity and disability in physically ill patients
- All patients with depression should be examined for suicidal ideation
- Depression is treatable in physically ill patients

Wells KB, Stewart A, Hays RD, Burnam MA, Rogers W, Daniels M, et al. The functioning and well-being of depressed patients. Results from the medical outcomes study. *JAMA* 1989;262:914-9

Carson AJ, Best S, Warlow C, Sharpe M. How common is suicidal ideation among neurology outpatients? *BMJ* 2000;320:1311-2

Gill D, Hatcher S. Antidepressants for depression in medical illness. *Cochrane Database Syst Rev* 2000;(4):CD001312

Further reading

- Kessler RC, McGonagle KA, Zhao S, Nelson CB, Hughes M, Eshleman S, et al. Lifetime and 12-month prevalence of DSM-IIIR psychiatric disorders in the United States: results of the national comorbidity survey. *Arch Gen Psychiatr* 1994;51,8-19
- Rodin G, Craven J, Littlefield C. *Depression in the medically ill: an integrated approach.* New York NY: Brunner/Mazel, 1991
- Royal College of Physicians, Royal College of Psychiatrists. *The psychological care of medical patients: recognition of need and service provision.* London: RCP, RCPsych, 1995

The diagram of the distribution of neurotic symptoms in the UK population is adapted from Jenkins et al *Psychol Med* 1997;27:765-74. The graph of association between depression and mortality after myocardial infarction. is adapted from Frasure Smith et al *JAMA* 1993;270: 1819-25. The diagram showing pathways to depression is adapted from Rodin et al *Depression in the medically ill* 1991. The meta-analysis of trials comparing antidepressants is adapted from Gill and Hatcher *Cochrane Database Syst Rev* 2000;(4):CD001312.

5 Anxiety in medical patients

Allan House, Dan Stark

Doctors often consider anxiety to be a normal response to physical illness. Yet, anxiety afflicts only a minority of patients and tends not to be prolonged. Any severe or persistent anxious response to physical illness merits further assessment.

What is anxiety?

Anxiety is a universal and generally adaptive response to a threat, but in certain circumstances it can become maladaptive. Characteristics that distinguish abnormal from adaptive anxiety include

- Anxiety out of proportion to the level of threat
- Persistence or deterioration without intervention (>3 weeks)
- Symptoms that are unacceptable regardless of the level of threat, including
  Recurrent panic attacks
  Severe physical symptoms
  Abnormal beliefs such as thoughts of sudden death
- Disruption of usual or desirable functioning.
  One way to judge whether anxiety is abnormal is to assess whether it is having a negative effect on the patient's functioning.
  Abnormal anxiety can present with various typical symptoms and signs, which include
- Autonomic overactivity
- Behaviours such as restlessness and reassurance seeking
- Changes in thinking, including intrusive catastrophic thoughts, worry, and poor concentration
- Physical symptoms such as muscle tension or fatigue.

Classification of abnormal anxiety

Abnormal anxiety can be classified according to its clinical features. In standardised diagnostic systems there are four main patterns of abnormal anxiety.

Anxious adjustment disorder—Anxiety is closely linked in time to the onset of a stressor.

Generalised anxiety disorder—Anxiety is more pervasive and persistent, occurring in many different settings.

Panic disorder—Anxiety comes in waves or attacks and is often associated with panicky thoughts (catastrophic thoughts) of impending disaster and can lead to repeated emergency medical presentations.

Phobic anxiety—Anxiety is provoked by exposure to a specific feared object or situation. Medically related phobic stimuli include blood, hospitals, needles, doctors and (especially) dentists, and painful or unpleasant procedures.

Additionally, anxiety often presents in association with depression. Mixed anxiety and depressive disorders are much more common than anxiety disorders alone. Treatment for the depression may resolve the anxiety. Anxiety can also be the presenting feature of other psychiatric illnesses common in physically ill people, such as delirium or drug and alcohol misuse.

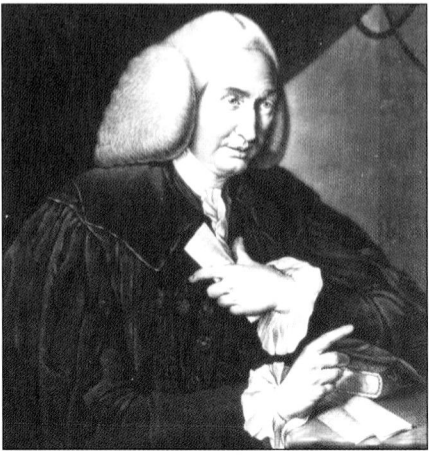

William Cullen (1710-90) coined the term neurosis (though the term as he used it bears little resemblance to modern concepts of anxiety disorders)

Somatic and psychological symptoms of anxiety disorders

In all anxiety disorders
- Palpitations, pounding heart, accelerated heart rate
- Trembling or shaking
- Difficulty in breathing
- Chest pain or discomfort
- Feeling dizzy, unsteady, faint, light headed
- Fear of losing control, going crazy, passing out
- Sweating
- Dry mouth
- Feeling of choking
- Nausea or abdominal discomfort
- Feeling that objects are unreal or that self is distant
- Fear of dying
- Numbness or tingling sensations
- Hot flushes or cold chills

In more severe or generalised anxiety disorders
- Muscle tension or aches and pains
- Feeling keyed up, on edge, or mentally tense
- Exaggerated response to minor surprises or being startled
- Persistent irritability
- Restlessness, inability to relax
- Sensation of difficulty swallowing, lump in the throat
- Difficulty concentrating or "mind going blank" from anxiety or worry
- Difficulty in getting to sleep because of worry

Distinguishing features of anxiety disorders

Anxious adjustment disorder
Prevalence in general population—Not known
Cardinal features
- Onset of symptoms within 1 month of an identifiable stressor
- No specific situation or response

Generalised anxiety disorder
Prevalence in general population—31 cases/1000 adults
Cardinal features
- Period of 6 months with prominent tension, worry, and feelings of apprehension about everyday problems
- Present in most situations and no specific response

Panic disorder
Prevalence in general population—8 cases/1000 adults
Cardinal features
- Discrete episode of intense fear or discomfort with crescendo pattern; starts abruptly and reaches a maximum in a few minutes
- Occurs in many situations, with a hurried exit the typical response

Phobia
Prevalence in general population—11 cases/1000 adults
Cardinal features
- No specific symptom pattern
- Occurs in specific situations, with an avoidance response

Detecting anxiety and panic

Who is at risk?—Certain groups are more vulnerable to anxiety disorders: younger people, women, those with social problems, and those with previous psychiatric problems. However, such associations are less consistent in the setting of life threatening illness, perhaps because susceptibility to anxiety becomes less important as the stressor becomes more severe. Pathological anxiety is commoner among patients with a chronic medical condition than in those without.

Excluding physical causes—There are many presentations with physical complaints whose aetiology may be due to anxiety. Equally, several physical illnesses can cause anxiety or similar symptoms. When such disorders cannot be reliably distinguished from anxiety by clinical examination they need to be excluded through appropriate investigation. A firm diagnosis of anxiety should therefore be made only when a positive diagnosis can be supported by the presence of a typical syndrome and after appropriate investigation.

Use of screening questionnaires—Screening, with self completed questionnaires, has been widely used to improve detection of psychiatric morbidity, including anxiety. Such questionnaires are acceptable to patients and can be amenable to computerised automation in the clinic. The hospital anxiety and depression scale, the general health questionnaire, and many quality of life instruments include anxiety items. No one questionnaire has been consistently shown to be preferable to another.

Iatrogenic anxiety—Anxiety symptoms can be caused by poor communication (see chapters 1 and 2) and by prescribed drugs. Well known causes include corticosteroids, β adrenoceptor agonists, and metoclopramide, but doctors should remember that many less commonly used drugs can cause psychiatric syndromes.

Treatment of anxiety and panic

General management

Treating anxiety is part of the management of most medical conditions. It can lead to direct improvement of symptoms or improve patient compliance. It is important to intervene if a positive diagnosis of anxiety is made. Without treatment, anxiety is associated with increased disability, increased use of health service resources, and impaired quality of life.

Involving a mental health professional is not always possible for anxious patients, particularly those in general hospital settings. The range of available services is often limited, and not all patients are prepared to accept referral. Since many patients have to be managed without recourse to psychiatric services, treating anxiety should be considered a core skill for all doctors.

Giving information is often the first step in helping anxious patients, so much so that it has been said that knowledge is reassurance. While information must be tailored to the wishes of the individual, many patients want more information than they are given. Such a simple step as showing people where they are to be cared for can reduce anxiety.

Effective communication is central to information giving, with evidence that anxiety is associated with poor communication. Training doctors to use open questions, discuss psychological issues, and summarise—and to avoid reassurance, "advice mode," and leading questions—has been shown to lead to greater disclosure and enduring change in patients with psychological problems.

Reassurance is one of the most widely practised clinical skills. Doctors often need to tell patients that their symptoms are not due to occult disease. Simple reassurance, however, may be

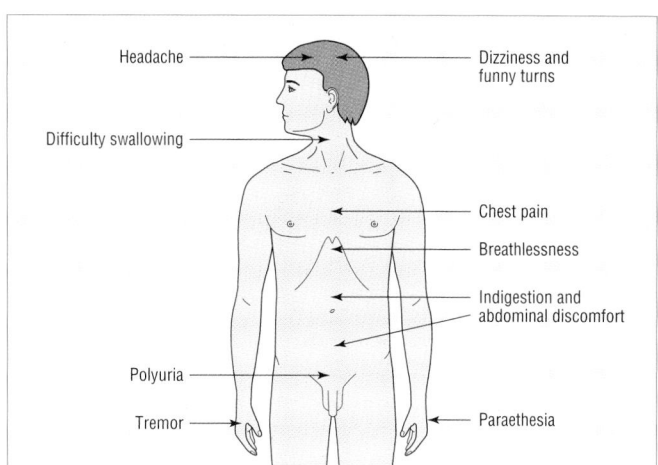

Common physical problems that may be caused by anxiety

Medical conditions mimicking or directly resulting in anxiety

- Poor pain control—Such as ischaemic heart disease, malignant infiltration
- Hypoxia—May be episodic in both asthma and pulmonary embolus
- Hypocapnia—May be due to occult bronchial hyperreactivity
- Central nervous system disorders (structural or epileptic)
- Anaemia
- Hypoglycaemia
- Hyperkalaemia
- Alcohol or drug withdrawal
- Vertigo
- Thyrotoxicosis
- Hypercapnia
- Hyponatraemia

Self reported questionnaires used to assess anxiety

Hospital anxiety and depression scale

Advantages
- Excludes somatic symptoms of disease
- Brevity (14 items in all, 7 concerning anxiety)
- Widespread use in cancer and other physical illnesses
- More effective than many other instruments
- Used as a screen and a measure of progress

Disadvantages
- Recent concern that, used alone, it is poor at detecting depression

State-trait anxiety inventory

Advantages
- Specific to anxiety
- Used as a screen and a measure of progress

Disadvantages
- Used alone does not detect depression
- Longer (20-40 items) than many other self reported questionnaires

General health questionnaire

Advantages
- Brevity (12 or 28 items)
- Excludes somatic symptoms of disease
- Used as a screen and a measure of progress

Disadvantages
- May not be accurate in detecting chronic problems

Common drug causes of anxiety

- Anticonvulsants—Carbamazepine, ethosuximide
- Antimicrobials—Cephalosporins, ofloxacin, aciclovir, isoniazid
- Bronchodilators—Theophyllines, β_2 agonists
- Digitalis—At toxic levels
- Oestrogen
- Insulin—When hypoglycaemic
- Non-steroidal anti-inflammatory drugs—Indomethacin
- Antidepressants—Specific serotonin reuptake inhibitors
- Antihistamines
- Calcium channel blockers—Felodipine
- Dopamine
- Inotropes—Adrenaline, noradrenaline
- Levodopa
- Corticosteroids
- Thyroxine

Many drugs can cause palpitation or tremor, but these should be easily distinguished from anxiety by clinical examination

ineffective for anxious patients; their anxiety may be reduced initially by the consultation, but it rapidly returns. Several theoretical models of this problem have been suggested, based on the patterns of thinking ("cognitions") of people who are difficult to reassure.

Preparation for unpleasant procedures can remove the additional burden of facing the unknown. It may also allow planning of short term tactics for dealing with anxiety provoking circumstances. Anxious patients are highly vigilant and overaware of threatening stimuli. They often use "quick fix" techniques based on avoidance of threat to reduce anxiety; such strategies are generally maladaptive and result in increasing disability. In some medical situations, however, such avoidance may not be a bad thing if the threat is temporary. A similar effect is seen with use of benzodiazepine to provide temporary relief from anxiety symptoms that will not recur because the stressor is not persistent.

Behavioural treatments are among the most effective treatments for anxiety disorders. Many patients restrict their activities in response to anxiety, which often has the effect of increasing both the level of anxiety and the degree of disability in the longer term. The principle of treatment is that controlled exposure to the anxiety producing stimulus will eventually lead to diminution in symptoms. Although specific behavioural treatments will normally be conducted by specialists, other clinicians should be aware of the basic principles. It is important to encourage and help patients to maintain their normal activities as much as possible, even if this causes temporary increases in anxiety.

Drug treatments—Several drugs can be used to treat anxiety, each with its own advantages and disadvantages. Long term benzodiazepine dependence and misuse are considered by many to be a problem in medical practice. Although the evidence for this is conflicting, the use of benzodiazepines may be reserved for the short term treatment of anxiety and for emergencies.

Drug withdrawal—Dependence on other substances, particularly analgesics and alcohol, occurs fairly frequently in the context of anxiety. This often results from self medication for anxiety. In this situation withdrawal from the existing "treatment" will be an important part of the anxiety management programme.

Role of specialist psychological treatment

Clinical studies indicate that psychological interventions for anxiety can be effective both in general psychiatric settings and for physically ill patients. The most popular, and those with the best evidence to support them, are based on the principles of behaviour, cognitive behaviour, or interpersonal therapy.

In behaviour and cognitive behaviour therapies the main aim is to help patients identify and challenge unhelpful ways of thinking about and coping with physical symptoms and their meaning, about themselves, and about how they should live their lives. In interpersonal therapies the main focus is on relationships with family members and friends—how such relationships are affected by illness and how they influence patients' current emotional state. Patients need to know that such therapies may be both brief and practical. Fewer than six sessions may be enough, concentrating on symptoms or the immediate problems associated with them and learning new ways of dealing with problems. In only a minority of cases is more extended therapy needed, usually when anxiety is longer standing and only partially due to associated physical disease.

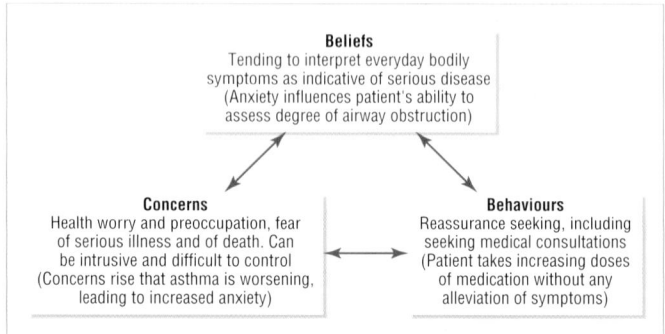

Characteristic features of health anxiety (using the example of asthma)

Drug interventions in anxious medical patients

β Blockers
- Benefits unproved in randomised controlled trials
- Help to control palpitation and tremor, but not anxiety itself
- Often used for performance anxiety, such as in interviews or examinations

Tricyclic antidepressants (such as imipramine)
- Likely to be beneficial (number needed to treat = 3)
- Anxiolytic effect is slow in onset (weeks)
- Not dependency inducing
- Useful in panic disorder or in anxiety with depression
- Anticholinergic effects can be ameliorated by a low starting dose

Selective serotonin reuptake inhibitors (such as sertraline)
- Benefit unproved but suggested
- Less anticholinergic effects than tricyclic antidepressants
- Start at low dose in anxious patients

Short acting benzodiazepines (such as alprazolam)
- Effectiveness and relative lack of toxicity well established
- All benzodiazepines can induce dependency
- Rapid onset of effect, but problems may recur on withdrawal
- Less likely to accumulate in liver

Antipsychotics (such as haloperidol)
- Benefits unproved in randomised controlled trials
- Useful adjunct to benzodiazepines
- Less respiratory depression that benzodiazepines
- Not dependency inducing
- Risk of acute dystonia, akathisia, and parkinsonism
- Avoid long term use because of risk of tardive dyskinesia

Buspirone
- Limited evidence for effectiveness from randomised controlled trials, few clinicians are convinced
- Causes some nausea and dizziness

Further reading
- Noyes R, Hoehn-Saric R. Anxiety in the medically ill: disorders due to medical conditions and substances. In: Noyes R, Hoehn-Saric R, eds. *The anxiety disorders*. Cambridge: Cambridge University Press, 1998:285-334
- Colon EA, Popkin MK. Anxiety and panic. In: Rundell JR, Wise MG, eds. *Textbook of consultation-liaison psychiatry*. Washington DC: American Psychiatric Press, 1996:403-25
- Westra HA, Stewart SH. Cognitive behavioural therapy and pharmacotherapy: complementary or contradictory approaches to the treatment of anxiety? *Clin Psychol Rev* 1998;18:307-40
- Cochrane Depression Anxiety and Neurosis Group. See list of reviews at www.update-software.com/abstracts/g240index.htm

6 Functional somatic symptoms and syndromes

Richard Mayou, Andrew Farmer

Concern about symptoms is a major reason for patients to seek medical help. Many of the somatic symptoms that they present with—such as pain, weakness, and fatigue—remain unexplained by identifiable disease even after extensive medical assessment. Several general terms have been used to describe this problem—somatisation, somatoform, abnormal illness behaviour, medically unexplained symptoms, and functional symptoms. We will use the term functional symptoms, which does not assume psychogenesis but only a disturbance in bodily functioning.

Classification of functional syndromes

Most functional symptoms are transient, but a sizeable minority become persistent. Persistent symptoms are often multiple and disabling and may be described as functional syndromes. Although different medical and psychiatric classifications of functional syndromes exist, these are simply alternative ways of describing the same conditions.

Medical syndromes (such as fibromyalgia and chronic fatigue, chronic pain, and irritable bowel syndromes) highlight patterns of somatic symptoms, often in relation to particular bodily systems. Although they are useful in everyday medical practice, recent studies show there is substantial overlap between them.

Psychiatric syndromes (such as anxiety, depression, and somatoform disorders) highlight psychological processes and the number of somatic symptoms irrespective of the bodily system to which they refer. Depression and anxiety often present with somatic symptoms that may resolve with effective treatment of these disorders. In other cases the appropriate psychiatric diagnostic category is a somatoform disorder.

The existence of parallel classificatory systems is confusing. Both have merits, and both are imperfect. For many functional symptoms, a simple description of the symptom qualified with the descriptors single or multiple and acute or chronic may suffice. When diagnosis of a functional syndrome seems appropriate a combination of medical and psychiatric descriptors conveys the most information, such as "irritable bowel syndrome with anxiety disorder."

A major obstacle to effective management is patients feeling disbelieved by their doctor. Patients who present with symptoms that are not associated with disease may be thought by some to be "putting it on." The deliberate manufacture of symptoms or signs, however, is probably rare in ordinary practice.

Epidemiology

Community based studies report annual prevalences of 6-36% for individual troublesome symptoms. In primary care only a small proportion of patients presenting with such symptoms ever receive a specific disease diagnosis. The World Health Organization found functional symptoms to be common and disabling in primary care patients in all countries and cultures studied. Up to half of these patients remain disabled by their symptoms a year after presentation, the outcome being worse for those referred to secondary and tertiary care. The clinical and public health importance of functional symptoms has been greatly underestimated.

Some common functional symptoms and syndromes

- Muscle and joint pain (fibromyalgia)
- Low back pain
- Tension headache
- Atypical facial pain
- Chronic fatigue
- Non-cardiac chest pain
- Palpitation
- Non-ulcer dyspepsia
- Irritable bowel
- Dizziness
- Insomnia

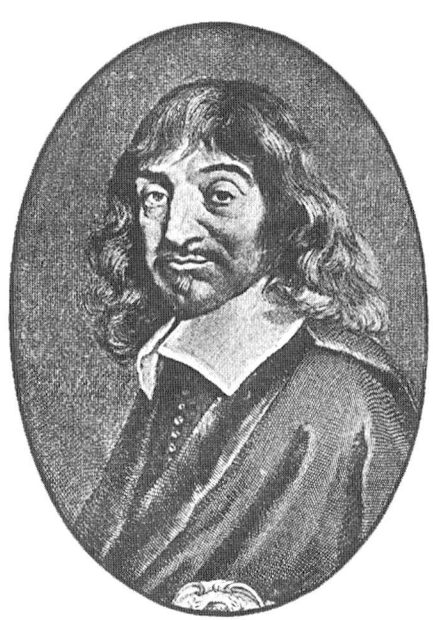

René Descartes, who formulated the philosophical principle of separation of brain and mind. This has led to continuing dualism—separation of body and mind—in Western medicine and difficulty in accepting the interaction of physical and psychological factors in aetiology

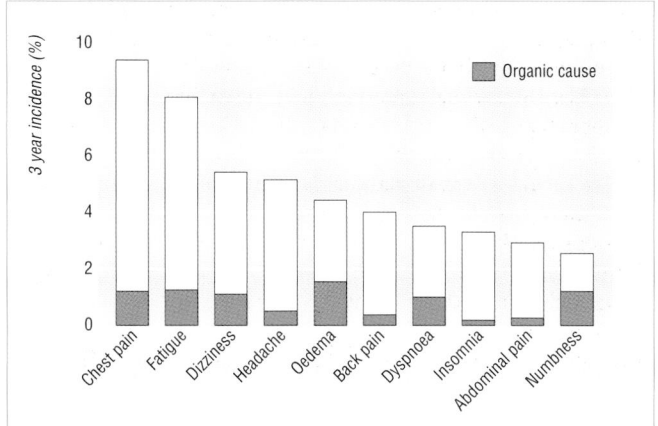

Three year incidence of 10 common presenting symptoms and proportion of symptoms with a suspected organic cause in US primary care

Causal factors

The cause of functional symptoms and syndromes is not fully understood, and it is therefore best to remain neutral regarding aetiological theories. In practice, functional symptoms are often attributed to single cause, which may be pathological (such as "a virus") or psychological (such as "stress"). This simplistic and dualistic approach is unhelpful both in explaining the cause to a patient and in planning treatment. The available evidence suggests that biological, psychological, interpersonal, and healthcare factors are all potentially important.

The dualistic, single factor view has tended to emphasise psychological over biological factors, as exemplified by the commonly used term "somatisation." However, recent evidence suggests that biological factors (especially reversible functional disturbance of the nervous system) are relevant to many functional syndromes, as they are to depression and anxiety disorders. A pragmatic doctor therefore asks not whether symptoms are "physical" or "mental" but whether they are fixed or are reversible by appropriate intervention.

The role of interpersonal factors in general, and of doctors and the health system in particular, in exacerbating functional symptoms has received less attention than it deserves. Raising fears of disease, performing unnecessary investigations and treatments, and encouraging disability are probably common adverse effects of medical consultations. However, denying the reality of patients' symptoms may damage the doctor-patient relationship and drive patients from evidence based care into the arms of the unhelpful, unscientific, and unscrupulous.

Aetiological factors can also be usefully divided into the stage of illness at which they have their effect. That is, they may be predisposing, precipitating, or perpetuating. Predisposing and precipitating factors are useful in producing a fuller understanding of why a patient has the symptom, while perpetuating factors are the most important for treatment.

Precipitating factors—Symptoms may arise from an increased awareness of physiological changes associated with stress, depression, anxiety and sometimes disease and injury. They become important to the patients when they are severe and when they are associated with fears of, or belief in, disease.

Predisposing factors increase the chance that such symptoms will become important. Some people are probably biologically and psychologically predisposed to develop symptoms. Fear of disease may result from previous experience—for example, a middle aged man with a family history of heart disease is likely to become concerned about chest pain.

Perpetuating factors are those that make it more likely that symptoms and associated disability persists. Patients' understandable attempts to alleviate their symptoms may paradoxically exacerbate them. For example, excessive rest to reduce pain or fatigue may contribute to disability in the longer term. Doctors may also contribute to this by failing to address patients' concern or unwittingly increasing fear of disease (such as by excessive investigation). The provision of disability benefits can also be a financial disincentive for some patients to return to jobs they dislike, and the process of litigation may maintain a focus on disability rather than recovery.

Detection and diagnosis

Almost any symptom can occur in the absence of disease, but some, such as fatigue and subjective bloating, are more likely to be functional than others. Surprisingly, the more somatic symptoms a person has, the less likely it is that these symptoms reflect the presence of disease and the more likely there is associated depression and anxiety.

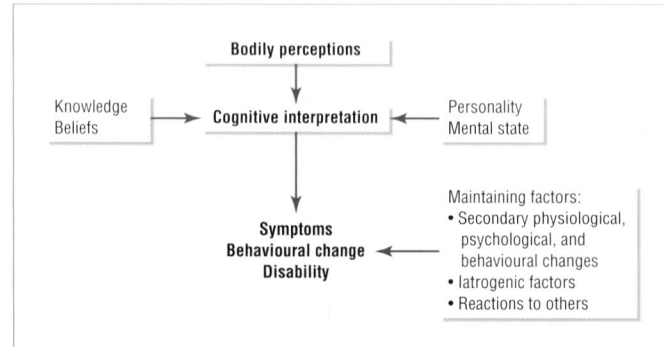

Interactive aetiology of "unexplained symptoms"

Iatrogenic factors in development of medically unexplained symptoms

- Appearance of uncertainty and inability to provide an explanation
- Expressed concern about disease explanations
- Failure to convince patient that the complaint is accepted as genuine
- Reassurance without a positive explanation being given
- Ambiguous and contradictory advice
- Excessive investigation and treatment

Individualised aetiological formulation for patient with chronic pain

Causes	Predisposing factors	Precipitating factors	Perpetuating factors
Biological	Genetic?	Injury at work	Effect of immobility Physiological mechanisms
Psychological	Lack of care as child	Trauma	Fear of worsening pain Avoid activity
Interpersonal	Family history of illness Dissatisfaction with work	Response of employer	Oversolicitous care Litigation process
Medical system	—	Misleading explanation of pain	Focus solely on somatic problems

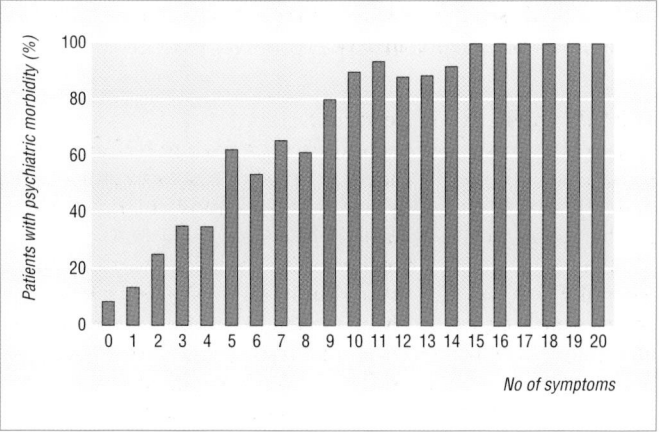

Association between number of unexplained physical symptoms and psychiatric disorder (anxiety and depression) in an international study of primary care attenders

Patients with functional symptoms can be detected by maintaining an awareness of the problem when seeing new patients and by the use of somatic symptom questionnaires (large numbers of symptoms are more likely to be functional).

Management

Although it is essential to consider disease as the cause of the patient's symptoms an approach exclusively devoted to this can lead to difficulties if none is found. Making explicit from the start the possibility that the symptoms may turn out to be functional keeps the option of a wider discussion open. Even if more specialist treatment is needed, then the problem has, from the outset, been framed in a way that enables psychological treatment to be presented as part of continuing medical care rather than as an unacceptable and dismissive alternative. In this way it is possible to avoid an anxious disabled patient being treated by a bewildered frustrated doctor.

Investigation
An appropriate physical examination and necessary medically indicated investigation are clearly essential. Thereafter, before further investigation is done, the potential adverse psychological effect on the patient should be balanced against the likelihood and value of new information that may be obtained.

Reassurance and explanation
Most patients are reassured by being told that the symptoms they have are common and rarely associated with disease and that their doctor is familiar with them. This is especially so if accompanied by the promise of further review should the symptoms persist.

Reassurance needs to be used carefully, however. It is essential to elicit patients' specific concerns about their symptoms and to target reassurance appropriately. The simple repetition of bland reassurance that fails to address patients' fears is ineffective. If patients have severe anxiety about disease (hypochondriasis) repeated reassurance is not only ineffective but may even perpetuate the problem.

A positive explanation for symptoms is usually more helpful that a simple statement that there is no disease. Most patients will accept explanations that include psychological and social factors as well as physiological ones as long as the reality of symptom is accepted. The explanation can usefully show the link between these factors—for example, how anxiety can lead to physiological changes in the autonomic nervous system that cause somatic symptoms, which, if regarded as further evidence of disease, lead to more anxiety.

Further non-specialist treatment
A minority of patients need more than simple reassurance and explanation. Treatment should address patients' illness fears and beliefs, reduce anxiety and depression, and encourage a gradual return to normal activities.

There is good evidence that antidepressants often help, even when there are no clear symptoms of depression. Practical advice is needed, especially on coping effectively with symptoms and gradually returning to normal activity and work. Other useful interventions include help in dealing with major personal, family, or social difficulties and involving a close relative in management. Other members of the primary care or hospital team may be able to offer help with treatment, follow up, and practical help.

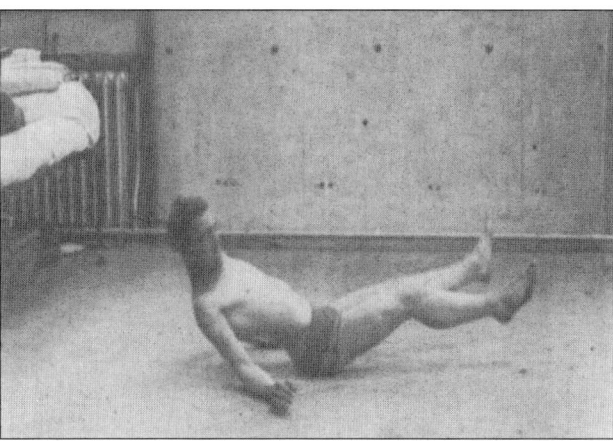

Functional somatic symptoms were common after combat in the first world war, such as this soldier's "hysterical pseudohypertrophic muscular spasms." The course and outcome of such symptoms can now be seen to have been substantially determined by varied medical and military approaches to prevention and treatment

---

Principles of assessment

- Identify patients' concerns and beliefs
- Review history of functional symptoms
- Explicitly consider both disease and functional diagnoses
- Appropriate medical assessment with explanation of findings
- Ask questions about patients' reaction to and coping with symptoms
- Use screening questions for psychiatric and social problems
- Consider interviewing relatives

Principles of treatment

- Explain that the symptoms are real and familiar to doctor
- Provide a positive explanation, including how behavioural, psychological, and emotional factors may exacerbate physiologically based somatic symptoms
- Offer opportunity for discussion of patient's and family's worries
- Give practical advice on coping with symptoms and encourage return to normal activity and work
- Identify and treat depression and anxiety disorders
- Discuss and agree a treatment plan
- Follow up and review

Non-specialist specific treatments

- Provide information and advice
- Agree a simple behavioural plan with patient and family
- Give advice about anxiety management
- Encourage use of diaries
- Advise about graded increase in activities
- Prescribe antidepressant drug
- Explain use of appropriate self help programmes

Specialist treatments

- Full and comprehensive assessment and explanation based on specialist assessment
- Cognitive behaviour therapy
- Supervised programme of graded increase in activity
- Antidepressants when these were previously not accepted or ineffective
- Illness specific interventions (such as rehabilitation programme for chronic pain)

Referral for specialist treatment

There is always a temptation to refer difficult patients to another doctor. However, this can result in greater long term difficulties if not carefully planned. When there is a good reason for further medical or psychiatric referral, then a clear explanation to the patient of the reason and an appropriately worded referral letter are essential.

Psychiatric treatments that may be required include more complex antidepressant drug regimens and specialist psychological interventions. Cognitive behaviour therapy has been shown to be effective in randomised controlled trials for a variety of functional syndromes (such as non-cardiac chest pain, irritable bowel, chronic pain, and chronic fatigue) and for patients with hypochondriasis.

Functional symptoms accompanying disease

Functional symptoms are also common in those who also have major disease. For example, after a heart attack or cardiac surgery, minor muscular chest aches and pains may be misinterpreted as evidence of angina, leading to unnecessary worry and disability. Explanation and advice, perhaps in the context of a cardiac rehabilitation programme, may make a substantial contribution to patients' quality of life.

Conclusion

An understanding of the interaction of biological, psychological, interpersonal, and medical factors in the predisposition, precipitation, and perpetuation of functional somatic symptoms allows convincing explanations to provided for patients and effective treatment to be planned.

Important components of general management include effective initial reassurance, a positive explanation, and practical advice. It is also important to identify early those who are not responding and who require additional specific interventions.

The difficulty that health systems have in effectively dealing with symptoms that are not attributable to disease reflects both intellectual and structural shortcomings in current care. The most salient of these is the continuing influence of mind-body dualism on our education and provision of care. In the longer term, scientific developments will break down this distinction. For the time being, it places primary care in a pivotal role in ensuring appropriate care for these patients.

The graph of incidence of common presenting symptoms in US primary care is adapted from Kroenke and Mangelsdorff, *Am J Med* 1989:86: 262-6. The graph of association between number of unexplained physical symptoms and psychiatric disorder is adapted from Kisely et al, *Psychol Med* 1997;27:1011-9. The picture of a shellshocked soldier is reproduced with permission of British Pathe. The graph of effects of cognitive behaviour treatment for hypochondriasis is adapted from Clark DM et al, *Br J Psychiatry* 1998;173:218-25.

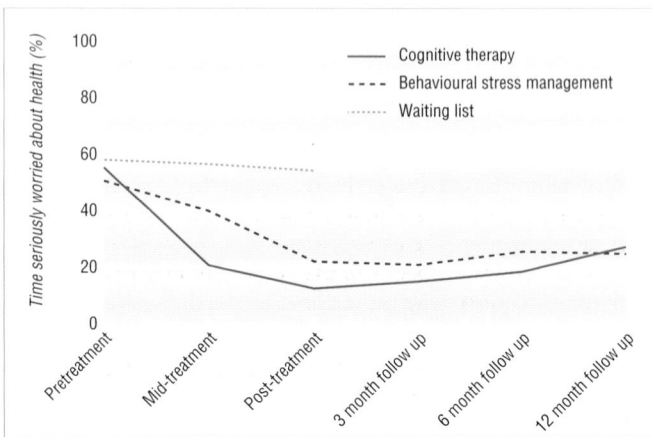

Randomised controlled trial of cognitive and behavioural treatments for hypochondriasis

---

Evidence based summary points

- Functional somatic symptoms are common in primary care in all countries and cultures
- Cognitive behaviour therapies are of general applicability
- Antidepressants are of value whether or not patient is depressed

Gureje O, Simon GE, Ustun TB, Goldberg DP. Somatization in cross-cultural perspective: a World Health Organization study in primary care. *Am J Psychiatry* 1997;154:989-95

Kroenke K, Swindle R. Cognitive-behavioral therapy for somatization and symptom syndromes: a critical review of controlled clinical trials. *Psychother Psychosom* 2000;69:205-15

O'Malley PG, Jackson JL, Santoro J, Tomkins G, Balden E, Kroenke K. Antidepressant therapy for unexplained symptoms and symptom syndromes. *J Fam Pract* 1999;48:980-90

Further reading

- Kroenke K, Mangelsdorff D. Common symptoms in ambulatory care: incidence, evaluation, therapy and outcome. *Am J Med* 1989;86: 262-6
- Mayou R, Bass C, Sharpe M. *Treatment of functional somatic symptoms.* Oxford: Oxford University Press, 1995
- Sharpe M, Carson AJ. "Unexplained" somatic syndromes, somatisation: do we need a paradigm shift? *Ann Intern Med* 2001;134:296
- Wessely S, Nimnuan C, Sharpe M. Functional somatic syndromes: one or many? *Lancet* 1999;354:936-9

7 Chronic multiple functional somatic symptoms

Christopher Bass, Stephanie May

The previous article in this series described the assessment and management of patients with functional somatic symptoms. Most such patients make no more than normal demands on doctors and can be helped with the approach outlined. However, a minority have more complex needs and require additional management strategies. These patients typically have a longstanding pattern of presenting with various functional symptoms, have had multiple referrals for investigation of these, and are regarded by their doctors as difficult to help.

Terminology

Because such patients may evoke despair, anger, and frustration in doctors, they may be referred to as "heartsink patients," "difficult patients," "fat folder patients," and "chronic complainers." The use of these terms is inadvisable. If patients read such descriptions in their medical notes they are likely to be offended and lose faith in their doctor and may make a complaint. In psychiatric diagnostic classifications these patients are often referred to as having somatisation disorder. We prefer the term "chronic multiple functional symptoms" (CMFS).

Epidemiology and detection

The prevalence of CMFS depends upon the number of different symptoms required for diagnosis and on the setting. Whilst each primary care doctor will have an average of 10-15 of such patients, they are more common in specialist medical settings where they may account for as many as 10% of referrals.

Most patients with CMFS are women. They often have recurrent depressive disorder and a longstanding difficulty with personal relationships and may misuse substances. There is an association with an emotionally deprived childhood and childhood physical and sexual abuse. Some patients will clearly have general disturbances of personality.

The risk of iatrogenic harm from over-investigation and over-prescribing for somatic complaints makes it important that patients with CMFS are positively identified and their management planned, usually in primary care. Potential CMFS patients may be identified simply by the thickness of their paper notes, from records of attendance and hospital referral, and by observation of medical, nursing, or clerical staff.

Management in primary care

Assessment
It is helpful if one doctor is identified as a patient's principal carer. Once a patient is identified as possibly having CMFS a systematic assessment is desirable. The case notes should be reviewed and the patient seen for one or more extended consultations.

Case notes—Patients with CMFS often have extensive case notes. Unless these are reviewed, much potentially useful information may remain hidden. It is also helpful to compile a summary of these records and to evaluate critically the accuracy of any previously listed complaints and diagnoses. The summary should include key investigations performed to date and any information about patients' personal and family circumstances.

Long appointment—During one or more long appointment a patient's current problems and history should be fully explored.

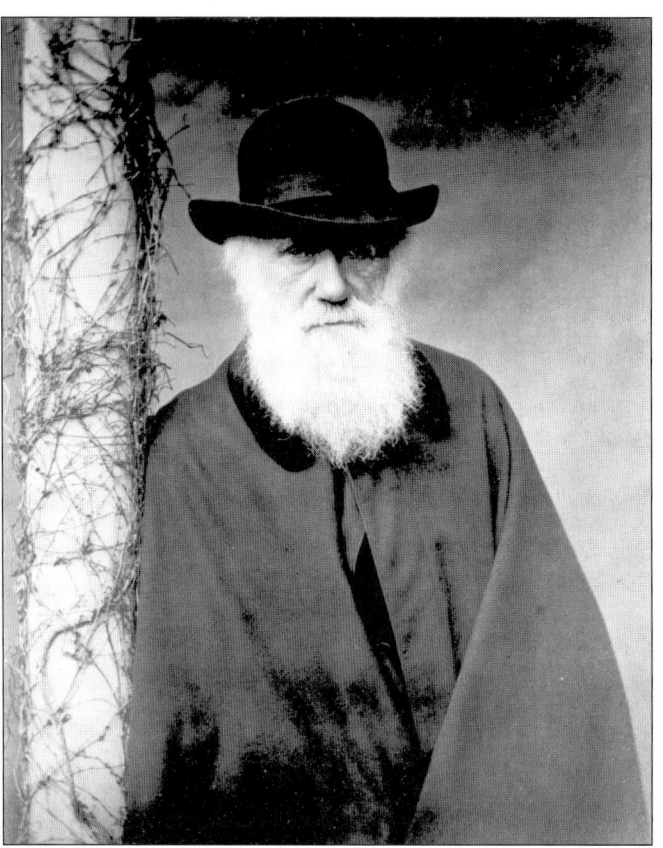

Charles Darwin (1809-82) suffered from chronic anxiety and varied physical symptoms that began shortly after his voyage in the *Beagle* to South America (1831-6). Despite many suggested medical explanations, these symptoms, which disabled him for the rest of his life and largely confined him to his home, remain medically unexplained

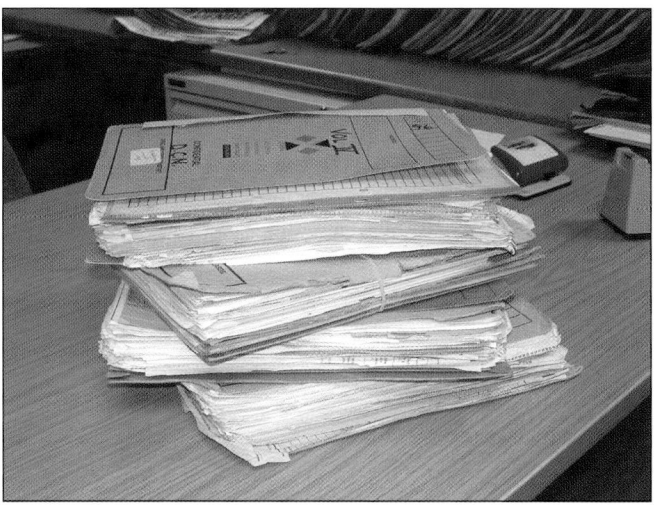

"Fat files" are a simple indicator of a high level of contact with medical services, which may indicate multiple chronic functional somatic complaints

Patients should be encouraged to talk not only about their symptoms but also about their concerns, emotional state, and social situation and the association of these with their symptoms. At the end of the assessment, patient and doctor should agree a current problem list, which can then be recorded in the notes.

Management

The initial long interviews serve not only to derive a problem list but also to foster a positive relationship between doctor and patient. Thereafter, the doctor should arrange to see the patient at regular, though not necessarily frequent, fixed intervals. These consultations should not be contingent on the patient developing new symptoms. Consultation outside these times should be discouraged.

Planned review

All symptoms reported by patients during these consultations must be acknowledged as valid. A detailed review of symptoms enhances the doctor-patient relationship and minimises the likelihood of missing new disease.

Reassurance that "nothing is wrong" may be unhelpful, possibly because a patient's aim may be to develop an understanding relationship with the doctor rather than relief of symptoms. Focused physical examination can be helpful, but there is a risk of patients receiving multiple diagnostic tests and referrals to specialists, and these should be minimised. Patients also often accumulate unnecessary prescribed drugs, and if so these should be reduced gradually over time.

If a satisfactory rapport can be established with a patient, new information about his or her emotional state, relationship difficulties, or childhood abuse may be revealed. In such cases the doctor may need to offer the patient a further long appointment to reassess the need for specialist psychological care.

Support for doctors

General practitioners managing patients with CMFS should arrange ongoing support for themselves, perhaps from a partner or another member of the primary care team with whom they can discuss their patients. A doctor and, for example, a practice nurse can jointly manage some of these patients if there is an agreed management plan and clear communication.

Referral to psychiatric services

Not all doctors will consider that they have the necessary skills or time to manage these patients effectively. Review by an appropriate specialist can then be helpful. Unfortunately, the decline in the number of "general physicians" and specialist mental health services' increasing focus on psychotic illness mean there are few appropriate specialists to refer to.

If referral is sought two questions must be considered: "Are there any local and appropriate psychiatric services?" and "How can I prepare the patient for this referral?" If available, liaison psychiatry services are often the most appropriate and experienced in this area of practice. To prepare the patient, a discussion emphasising the distressing nature of chronic illness and the expertise of the services in this area, together with a promise of continuing support from the primary care team, can help to make the referral seem less rejecting. If possible, the psychiatrist should visit the practice or medical department and conduct a joint consultation.

Assessment of chronic multiple functional somatic symptoms

- Elicit a history of the current complaints, paying special attention to recent life events
- Find out what the patient has been told by other doctors (as well as friends, relatives, and alternative practitioners). Does this accord with the medical findings?
- Elicit an illness history that addresses previous experience of physical symptoms and contact with medical services (such as illness as a child, illness of parents and its impact on childhood development, operations, time off school and sickness absence)
- Explore psychological and interpersonal factors in patient's development (such as quality of parental care, early abusive experiences, psychiatric history)
- Interview a partner or reliable informant (this may take place, consent permitting, in the patient's presence)
- After the interview attempt a provisional formulation

Useful interviewing skills for doctors managing patients with multiple physical complaints

- Adopt a flexible interviewing style—"I wonder if you've thought of it like this?"
- Try to remind the patient that physical and emotional symptoms often coexist—"I'm struck by the fact that, in addition to the fatigue, you've also been feeling very low and cannot sleep"
- Try "reframing" the physical complaints to indicate important temporal relationship between emergence of patient's somatic and emotional symptoms and relevant life events
- Respond appropriately to "emotional" cues such as anger
- Explore patient's illness beliefs and worst fears—"What is your worst fear about this pain?"

Management strategy for patients with chronic multiple functional somatic symptoms

- Try to be proactive rather than reactive—Arrange to see patients at regular, fixed intervals, rather than allowing them to dictate timing and frequency of visits
- During appointments, aim to broaden the agenda with patients—This involves establishing a problem list and allowing patients to discuss relevant psychosocial problems
- Stop or reduce unnecessary drugs
- Try to minimise patients' contacts with other specialists or practitioners—This will reduce iatrogenic harm and make containment easier if only one or two practitioners are involved
- Try to co-opt a relative as a therapeutic ally to implement your management goals
- Reduce your expectation of cure and instead aim for containment and damage limitation
- Encourage patients (and yourself) to think in terms of coping and not curing

---

Explanations to the patient

Present patient's problems as a summary with an invitation to comment:

"So let me see if I've understood you properly: you have had a lot of pain in your abdomen, with bloating and distension for the past four years. You have been attending the (GP) surgery most weeks because you've been very worried about cancer (and about your husband leaving you). You also told me that these pains often occur when you are anxious and panicky, and at these times other physical complaints such as trembling and nausea occur.

"I'm struck by the fact that all these complaints began soon after you had a very frightening experience in hospital, when your appendix was removed and you felt that 'No one was listening to my complaints or pain.'

"Have I got that right, or is there anything I've left out?"

Summary of a 15 year "segment" of the life of a patient with chronic multiple functional somatic symptoms

Date (age)	Symptoms (life events)	Referral	Investigations	Outcome
1970 (18)	Abdominal pain	GP to surgical outpatients	Appendicectomy	Normal appendix
1973 (21)	Pregnant (boyfriend in prison)	GP to obstetrics and gynaecology outpatients	Termination of pregnancy	—
1975-7 (23-25)	Bloating, abdominal pain, blackouts (stressful divorce)	GP to gastroenterology and neurology outpatients	All tests normal	Diagnosis of irritable bowel syndrome and unexplained syncope. Treated with fibre
1979 (27)	Pelvic pain (wants to be sterilised)	GP to obstetrics and gynaecology outpatients	Sterilised, ovaries preserved	Pelvic pain persists for 2 years after surgery
1981 (29)	Fatigue (problems at work)	GP to infectious disease clinic	Nothing abnormal detected	Diagnosis of myalgic encephalomyelitis made by patient. Joins self help group
1983 (31)	Aching, painful muscles	GP to rheumatology clinic	Mild cervical spondylosis. No treatment	Treated with amitriptyline 50 mg on referral to pain clinic. Some improvement
1985 (34)	Chest pain and breathlessness (son truanting from school)	Accident and emergency to chest clinic	Nothing abnormal detected, probable hyperventilation	Refer to psychiatric services

Specialist assessment

Before interviewing a patient, it is useful to request both the general practice and hospital notes and summarise the medical history. A typed summary of the "illness history" can be kept as a permanent record in the notes. This summary can guide future management and is especially useful when a patient is admitted subsequently as an emergency or when the receiving doctor has no prior knowledge of the patient.

Several important interviewing skills should be used during the assessment. These skills can be learnt using structured role playing and video feedback. They form the basis of a technique called reattribution, which has been developed to help the management of patients with functional somatic symptoms.

Specialist management

If a patient can understand and agree an initial shared formulation of the problems, an important first stage is reached. From this a plan of management can be negotiated. It is best to adopt a collaborative approach rather than a didactic or paternalistic manner. If it is difficult to arrive at an understanding of why the patient developed these symptoms at this particular time, then an alternative approach may have to be adopted. In essence this involves the doctor attempting to address those factors that are maintaining the symptoms.

Assessment and management go hand in hand. One of the main aims of management is to modify patients' often unrealistic expectations of the medical profession and to remind them of the limits to medicine. In many cases hopes may have been falsely raised, and patients expect either a cure or at least a considerable improvement in symptoms. Although this is desirable, it may not be attainable. Instead, the doctor should attempt to broaden the agenda, with an emphasis on helping patients to address personal concerns and life problems as well as somatic complaints. It is also necessary to encourage them to concentrate on coping rather than seeking a cure.

This process requires patience, and a capacity to tolerate frustration and setbacks. It may require several discussions in which the same issues are reviewed. In the long term, however, it can be rewarding for both patient and doctor.

Common problems in management

Management may be complicated by various factors. Firstly, preoccupation and anxious concern about symptoms may lead patients to make unhelpful demands of their doctor, which prove difficult to resist.

What is the cause of functional somatic symptoms?

- A variety of biological, psychological, and social factors have been shown to be associated with functional symptoms; the contribution of these factors will vary between patients
  Recent developments in neuroscience show altered functioning of the nervous system associated with functional symptoms, making the labelling of these as "entirely psychological" increasing inappropriate
- With our current knowledge, it is best to maintain "aetiological neutrality" about the cause of functional symptoms
- The main task of treatment is to identify those factors that may be maintaining a patient's symptoms and disability

Maintaining factors that should be focus of treatment in patients with multiple somatic symptoms

- Depression, anxiety, or panic disorder
- Chronic marital or family discord
- Physical inactivity
- Occupational stress
- Abnormal illness beliefs
- Iatrogenic factors
- Pending medicolegal and insurance claims

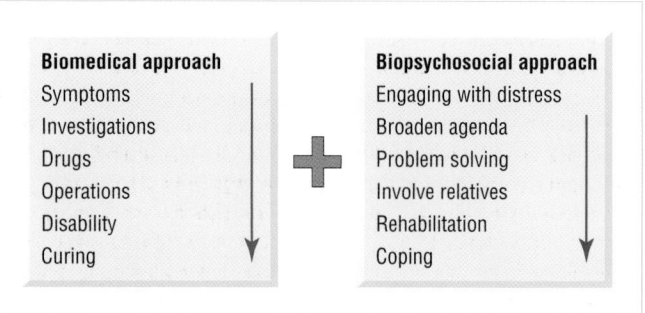

The aim of treatment for patients with chronic multiple functional symptoms is to add a biopsychosocial perspective to the existing biomedical approach

Secondly, there may be evidence of longstanding interpersonal difficulties, as indicated by remarks such as "Nobody cares" or "It's disgusting what doctors can do to you." Such comments may suggest that the patient's relationship with the doctor may reflect poor quality parental care or emotional deprivation in childhood. They are important for two reasons: firstly, the doctor may take these remarks personally, become demoralised or angry, and retaliate, which will destroy the doctor-patient relationship; and, secondly, the attitudes revealed may require more detailed psychological exploration.

Finally, iatrogenic factors may intervene that are beyond the treating doctor's control. Because these patients have often visited several specialists, conventional and alternative, they may have been given inappropriate information and advice, inappropriate treatment, or, in some cases, frank misdiagnosis.

Factitious disorders and malingering

Factitious disorders

Factitious disorders are characterised by feigned physical or psychological symptoms and signs presented with the aim of receiving medical care. They are therefore different from functional symptoms. The judgment that a symptom is produced intentionally requires direct evidence and exclusion of other causes. Most patients with factitious disorders are women with stable social networks, and more than half of these work in medically related occupations. Once factitious disorder is diagnosed, it is important to confront the patient but remain supportive. When factitious disorder is established in a person working in health care it is advisable to organise a multidisciplinary meeting involving the patient's general practitioner, a physician and surgeon, a psychiatrist, and a medicolegal representative.

If, and only if, the deliberate feigning of symptoms and signs can be established (such as by observation of self mutilation) should patients be confronted. It is helpful if both a psychiatrist and the referring doctor (who should have met to discuss the aims, content, and possible outcomes of the meeting beforehand) can carry out the confrontation jointly. This "supportive confrontation" is done by gently but firmly telling the patient that you are aware of the role of their behaviour in the illness whilst at the same time offering psychological care to help with this. After confrontation, patients usually stop the behaviour or leave the clinic. Only sometimes do they engage in the psychiatric care offered.

Malingering

A distinction should be made between factitious disorders and malingering. Malingerers deliberately feign symptoms to achieve a goal (such as to avoid imprisonment or gain money). Malingering is behaviour and not a diagnosis. The extent to which a doctor feels it necessary to confront this issue will depend on the individual circumstances.

Conclusion

Patients with multiple longstanding functional symptoms are relatively uncommon, but their interaction with the health system is memorable in that it often leaves both them and their doctors frustrated. Their effective management requires that special attention be paid to their interpersonal difficulties (including those arising in their relationship with the doctor), the limiting of unhelpful demands, and the avoidance of iatrogenic harm. As with any chronic illness, confident management and getting to know a patient as a person can change what is often a frustrating task into a rewarding one.

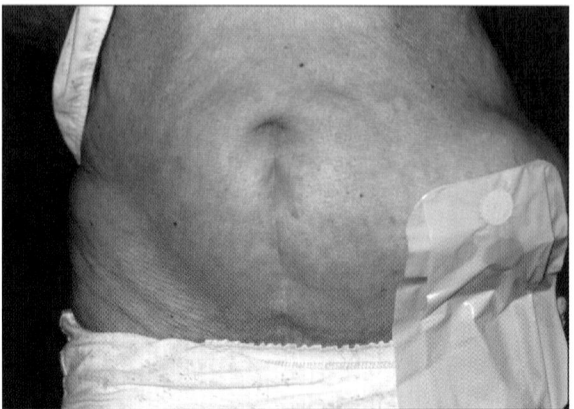

Failing to recognise and institute appropriate management for patients with multiple functional somatic symptoms may lead to iatrogenic harm from excessive and inappropriate medical and surgical intervention

---

Münchausen's syndrome

- Münchausen's syndrome is an uncommon subtype of factitious illness in which the patient, who is often a man with sociopathic traits and an itinerant lifestyle, has a long career of attending multiple hospitals with factitious symptoms and signs
- Management is as for factitious disorder, but engagement with psychiatric treatment is rare

---

Evidence based summary

- Prevalence of chronic multiple functional somatic symptoms depends on how many functional symptoms are required—the fewer symptoms the higher the prevalence
- Patients with chronic multiple functional somatic symptoms (somatisation disorder) can be effectively managed in primary care, with resulting cost savings

Kroenke K, Spitzer RL, deGruy FV, Hahn SR, Linzer M, Williams JB, et al. Multisomatoform disorder. An alternative to undifferentiated somatoform disorder for the somatizing patient in primary care. *Arch Gen Psychiatry* 1997;54:352-8

Smith GR, Monson RA, Ray DC. Psychiatric consultation in somatization disorder—a randomized controlled study. *N Engl J Med* 1986;314:1407-13

Suggested reading

- Bass C. Management of somatisation disorder. *Prescribers J* 1996;36:198-205
- Dixon DM, Sweeney KG, Pereira Gray DJ. The physician healer ancient magic or modern science? *Br J Gen Pract* 1999;49:309-12
- Fink P, Rosendal M, Toft T. Assessment and treatment of functional disorders in general practice: the extended reattribution and management model—an advanced educational program for nonpsychiatric doctors. *Psychosom* 2002;43:93-131
- Smith GR. Management of patients with multiple symptoms. In: Mayou R, Bass C, Sharpe M, eds. *Treatment of functional somatic symptoms*. Oxford: Oxford University Press, 1995:175-87
- Tate P. *The doctor's communication handbook*. Oxford: Radcliffe Medical Press, 1994

8 Cancer

Craig A White, Una Macleod

Cancer is the most feared of diseases. Unsurprisingly, it causes considerable psychological distress in patients, families, carers, and often those health professionals who care for them. Only a minority of cancer patients develop psychiatric illness, but other psychologically and socially determined problems are common. These include unpleasant symptoms such as pain, nausea, and fatigue; problems with finances, employment, housing, and childcare; family worries; and existential and spiritual doubts. Well planned care that fully involves patients and their families can minimise these problems.

Psychological consequences

Though often dismissed as "understandable," distress is a treatable cause of reduced quality of life and poorer clinical outcome. Some patients delay seeking help because they fear or deny their symptoms of distress. Presentation can be obvious, as depressed or anxious mood can manifest as increased severity of somatic complaints such as breathlessness, pain, or fatigue. Adjustment disorder is the commonest psychiatric diagnosis, and neuropsychiatric complications may occur. The risk of suicide is increased in the early stages of coping with cancer.

Depression
Depression is a response to perceived loss. A diagnosis of cancer and awareness of associated losses may precipitate feelings similar to bereavement. The loss may be of parts of the body (such as a breast or hair), the role in family or society, or impending loss of life. Severe and persistent depressive disorder is up to four times more common in cancer patients than in the general population, occurring in 10-20% during the disease.

Anxiety, fear, and panic
Anxiety is the response to a perceived threat. It manifests as apprehension, uncontrollable worry, restlessness, panic attacks, and avoidance of people and of reminders of cancer, together with signs of autonomic arousal. Patients may overestimate the risks associated with treatment and the likelihood of a poor outcome. Anxiety may also exacerbate or heighten perceptions of physical symptoms (such as breathlessness in lung cancer), and post-traumatic stress symptoms (with intrusive thoughts and avoidance of reminders of cancer) occasionally follow diagnosis or treatment that has been particularly frightening.

Certain cancers and treatments are associated with specific fears. Thus, patients with head and neck cancers may worry about being able to breathe and swallow. Patients may develop phobias and conditioned vomiting in relation to unpleasant treatments such as chemotherapy.

Neuropsychiatric syndromes
Delirium and dementia may arise from brain metastases, which usually originate from lung cancer but also from tumours of the breast and alimentary tract and melanomas. Brain metastases occasionally produce psychological symptoms before metastatic disease is discovered. Certain cancers (notably cancers of the lung, ovary, breast, or stomach and Hodgkin's lymphoma) sometimes produce neuropsychiatric problems in the absence of metastases (paraneoplastic syndromes). The aetiology is thought to be an autoimmune response to the tumour.

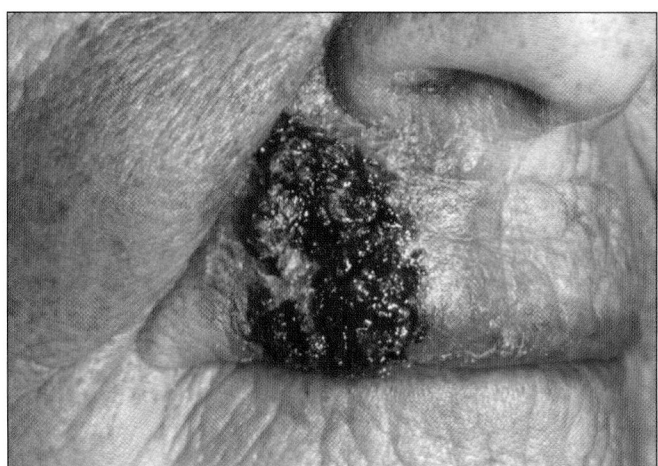

Squamous cell cascinoma on lip after radiotherapy. As well as the fear of cancer itself, an additional source of distress can be the potentially disfiguring nature of the disease and its treatment

> "Distress is an unpleasant emotional experience of a psychological, social, or spiritual nature that may interfere with a patient's ability to cope with cancer and its treatment. Distress extends along a continuum, ranging from common normal feelings of vulnerability, sadness, and fear to problems that can become disabling, such as depression, anxiety, panic, social isolation, and spiritual crisis"
>
> **US National Comprehensive Cancer Network**

Challenges faced by people with cancer
- Maintaining activity and independence
- Coping with treatment side effects
- Accepting cancer and maintaining a positive outlook
- Seeking and understanding medical information
- Regulating the feelings associated with cancer experiences
- Seeking support
- Managing stress

Who becomes distressed?

The severity of emotional distress is more closely related to a patient's pre-existing vulnerability than to the characteristics of the cancer. Distress is also more likely to occur at specific points in a patient's experience of cancer:

Diagnosis—Investigation and diagnosis are particularly stressful and can cause shock, anger, and disbelief as well as emotional distress. These resolve without intervention in most patients, but especially high levels of distress at this time are predictive of later emotional problems. It can help if doctors explain that patients' feelings are expected and normal ("I would expect you to have times when you feel tearful and cannot get it out of your head").

During treatment—Treatment itself can be a potent cause of distress. It may involve hospital attendance but also unpleasant surgery, radiotherapy, or chemotherapy. Side effects include hair loss and disfigurement. Patients worry about whether treatment is working and are likely to become distressed at times of apparent treatment failure.

End of treatment—At the end of apparently successful treatment some patients can experience "rebound" distress associated with the fear that the cancer might recur or spread. The ending of a prolonged relationship with the cancer service staff can lead to a sense of loss and vulnerability. It is only at this time that some patients become fully aware of the impact of their cancer experience.

After treatment—Like those with other life threatening illnesses, patients who survive cancer may reorder their life priorities and experience psychological benefits including a greater appreciation of some aspects of their life. Others need help to overcome continuing worries, including preoccupation with loss and illness, a tendency to avoid reminders of cancer, and difficulties coping with intimacy, return to work, and fears of recurrence. Fear of recurrence can manifest as a form of health anxiety with misinterpretation of physiological sensations (such as believing that pain associated with a muscle strain represents a recurrence of cancer) and the anxious seeking of reassurance.

Recurrence—Patients who believe they have been cured (that is, those most likely to be surprised by recurrence) are at greater risk of severe distress if recurrence occurs. Most patients report recurrence of cancer as more distressing than receiving the initial diagnosis.

Terminal disease—About 40% of people who develop cancer will die as a result. The terminal phase commonly brings fear of uncontrolled pain, of the process of dying, of what happens after death, and of the fate of loved ones. Depression is common in the terminal phase, especially in those with poorly controlled physical symptoms.

Management

People with cancer benefit from care in which psychological and medical care are coordinated. Apart from the obvious

---

Risk factors for psychiatric disorder

Patient
- History of psychiatric disorder
- Social isolation
- Dissatisfaction with medical care
- Poor coping (such as not seeking information or talking to friends)

Cancer
- Limitation of activities
- Disfiguring
- Poor prognosis

Treatment
- Disfiguring
- Isolating (such as bone marrow transplant)
- Side effects

Issues to be considered in planning care
- Patient's and family's understanding of the illness and its treatment
- Patient's and family's understanding of help available
- Explanation of how symptomatic relief will be provided
- How the patient can be fully involved in care
- Who will be managing the treatment plan
- Routine and emergency contact arrangements
- Practical help in everyday activities
- Support at home—role of hospital and residential care
- Involving and supporting family and friends

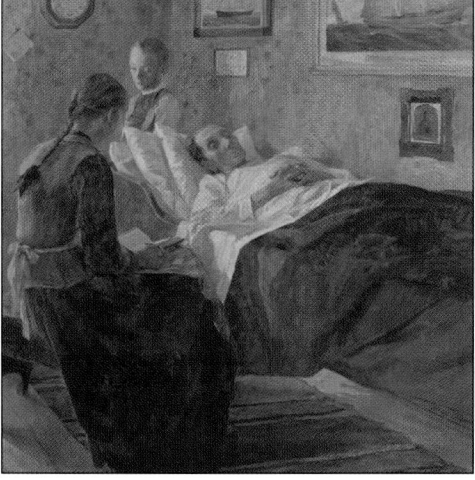

Depression is common in the terminal phase of cancer, especially in patients with poorly controlled physical symptoms (*Resignation* by Carl Wilhelm Wilhelmson (1866-1928))

Psychological care for cancer patients

In primary care
- Need for agreed local protocols
- Multidisciplinary skills and resources
- Individually agreed collaborative care for each patient
- Regular liaison with specialist units and local agencies
- Local training for all involved

In specialist units
- Training in psychological aspects of care for all staff
- Regular review of all individual treatment plans
- Protocols for routine management of "at risk" patients (such as relapse after chemotherapy)
- Involvement of specialist nurses and other staff with psychological expertise
- Access to psychiatrists and clinical psychologists with special interest in managing cancer problems for consultation and supervision
- Use of self help methods and voluntary agencies

benefits to quality of life, there is some evidence that encouraging an active approach to living with cancer can improve survival.

Most of the psychological care of cancer patients will be delivered in primary care. As for all chronic illness, a multidisciplinary approach and management protocols that include psychological as well as medical assessment and intervention are required. These protocols need not be specific for cancer as the issues are common to many medical conditions. The important point is that the staff involved have the skills to address psychological as well as medical problems. The danger is that psychological care can be neglected by the medical focus on cancer treatment. A case manager, whether nurse or doctor, who can coordinate the often diverse agencies involved in a cancer patient's care can ensure that treatment is delivered efficiently.

Assessment

Depressive and anxiety disorders are often unrecognised. There is therefore a need for active screening by simply asking patients about symptoms of anxiety and depression. A self rated questionnaire such as the hospital anxiety and depression scale (HADS) may be helpful. Doctors should be aware that patients may be distressed because of factors unrelated to cancer.

Treatment

Information—Doctors often underestimate the amount and frankness of information that most patients need and want. It is best given in a staged fashion with checks on patients' understanding and desire to hear more at each stage. Repetition and written information may be helpful. Summaries of agreed management plans have been found to improve patients' satisfaction and their adherence to medical treatment.

Social support—Most patients will receive this from family and friends. They may, however, not want to "burden others" and consequently may need encouragement to use this support by talking about their illness. Additional support can be provided by specific cancer related services such as the primary care team and specialist nurses.

Addressing worries—Staff often find it most difficult to help patients who talk about worries that reflect the reality of cancer (such as, "I am going to die"). It is important to do so because this may help planning and may reveal misconceptions, such as the inevitability of uncontrolled pain, that can then be addressed by giving accurate information about methods of pain control.

Managing anxiety—Accurate information (such as which physical symptoms are due to anxiety and which are due to cancer) and practical help are important. Anxious patients can be helped by relaxation strategies, including breathing exercises. Severe persistent anxiety may merit the short term prescription of anxiolytic drugs such as diazepam.

Managing depression—Depressive disorders should be managed in the same ways as they are in patients without cancer. Discussion, empathy, reassurance, and practical help are essential. Antidepressants have been shown to be effective in patients with cancer in randomised trials, although surprisingly few trials have been conducted. If in doubt about what drug to choose or about possible interactions with cancer treatment, it is important to check with a pharmacist. Specialist psychological intervention, such as formal cognitive-behavioural therapy, may also be required to treat persistent depression or anxiety.

Specialist referral

Structured psychological interventions (such as psycho-education and cognitive-behavioural based therapies)

Questions for assessing patients' anxiety and depression

- How are you feeling in yourself? Have you felt low or worried?
- Have you ever been troubled by feeling anxious, nervous, or depressed?
- What are your main concerns or worries at the moment?
- What have you been doing to cope with these? Has this been helpful?
- What effects do you feel cancer and its treatment will have on your life?
- Is there anything that would help you cope with this?
- Who do you feel you have helping you at the moment?
- Is there anyone else outside of the family?
- Have you any questions? Is there anything else you would like to know?

Principles of treatment

- Sympathetic interest and concern
- A clearly identified principal therapist who can coordinate all care
- Effective symptomatic relief
- Elicit and understand patient's beliefs and needs
- Collaborative planning of continuing care
- Information and advice—oral and written
- Involve patient in treatment decisions
- Involve family and friends
- Early recognition and treatment of psychological complications
- Clear arrangements to deal with urgent problems

Useful sources of information

- National Comprehensive Cancer Network. Distress management guidelines (www.nccn.org/physician_gls/index.html)
- National Cancer Institute. Cancer.gov (www.cancer.gov/cancer_information/)
- Cancer BACUP (www.cancerbacup.org.uk)
- Cancer Help UK (www.cancerhelp.org.uk/)
- Macmillan Cancer Relief (www.macmillan.org.uk/)
- Cancer Research UK (www.cancer.org.uk)
- International Psycho-Oncology Society (www.ipos-aspboa.org/iposnews.htm)

Specialist treatments

- Antidepressant drugs
- Effective drug treatment of pain, nausea, and other symptoms
- Problem solving discussion
- Cognitive-behavioural treatment of psychological complications
- Joint and family interviews to encourage discussion and planning
- Group support and treatment
- Cognitive-behavioural methods to help cope with chemotherapy and other unpleasant treatments

Referral decisions

- What specialist expertise in psycho-oncology is available at my local cancer centre or unit?
- What has helped when this patient has had problems before?
- Are there local cancer support groups that could help?
- Does this patient have problems that might benefit from specialist psychological or psychiatric intervention?
- Does this patient want to be referred to specialist services?
- Does this patient prefer individual or group based psychological intervention?

have been shown to reduce anxiety and depression in cancer patients and to improve adherence to medical treatment.

Patients with severe or persistent distress may need referral to an experienced clinical psychologist or psychiatrist. An increasing number of mental health professionals are attached to cancer centres and units, and other staff such as appropriately trained specialist nurses play an increasingly important role.

Increasing numbers of non-NHS agencies also offer psychological care for patients with cancer. When referring patients to such services it is important to check their quality and to ensure that their contribution is coordinated within an overall care plan.

The picture of skin cancer is reproduced with permission of Dr P Marazzi and Science Photo Library. *Resignation* is held at the Nationalmuseum, Stockholm, and is reproduced with permission of Bridgeman Art Library.

Evidence based summary

- Antidepressants are effective in treating depressed mood in cancer patients
- Cognitive-behavioural treatments are effective in relieving distress, especially anxiety, and in reducing disability
- Psychological interventions can be effective in relieving specific cancer related symptoms such as breathlessness

McDaniel JS, Musselman DL, Porter MR, Reed DA, Nemeroff CB. Depression in patients with cancer. Diagnosis, biology, and treatment. *Arch Gen Psychiatry* 1995;52:89-99

Sheard T, Maguire P. The effect of psychological interventions on anxiety and depression in cancer patients: results of two meta-analyses. *Br J Cancer* 1999;80:1770-80

Bredin M, Corner J, Krishnasamy M, Plant H, Bailey C, A'Hern R. Multicentre randomised controlled trial of nursing intervention for breathlessness in patients with lung cancer. *BMJ* 1999;318:901-4

Further reading

- Barraclough J. *Cancer and emotion : a practical guide to psycho-oncology.* 3rd ed. Chichester: John Wiley, 1998
- Burton M, Watson M. *Counselling patients with cancer.* Chichester: John Wiley, 1998
- Faulkener A, Maguire P. *Talking to cancer patients and their relatives.* Oxford: Oxford Medical Publications, 1994
- Holland JC. *Psycho-oncology.* Oxford: Oxford University Press, 1998
- Lewis S, Holland JC. *The human side of cancer: living with hope, coping with uncertainty.* London: Harper Collins, 2000
- Scott JT, Entwistle V, Sowden AJ, Watt I. Recordings or summaries of consultations for people with cancer. Cochrane Database of Systematic Reviews. 2001

9 Trauma

Richard Mayou, Andrew Farmer

Minor physical trauma is a part of everyday life, and for most people these injuries are of only transient importance, but some have psychiatric and social complications. Most people experience major trauma at some time in their lives.

Psychological, behavioural, and social factors are all relevant to the subjective intensity of physical symptoms and their consequences for work, leisure, and family life. As a result, disability may become greater than might be expected from the severity of the physical injuries.

Psychological and interpersonal factors also contribute to the cause of trauma, and clinicians should be alert to these and their implications for treatment. Tactful questioning, careful examination, and detailed record keeping are essential, especially for non-accidental injury by a patient or others:

- Ask for a detailed description of the cause of the incident
- Ask about previous trauma
- Ask about substance misuse—alcohol and drugs
- Look for patterns of injuries that may be non-accidental, deliberate self harm, or inflicted by others
- Check records
- If suspicious speak to other informants
- Discuss findings and suspicions with a colleague.

Dealing with the acute event

At a major incident it is important that members of the emergency services, especially ambulance staff and police, should seem calm and in control. This helps to relieve distress and prevent victims from suffering further injury. Explanation and encouragement can reduce fear at the prospect of being taken to hospital by ambulance. The needs of uninjured relatives and others involved should also be considered. Clearly recorded details of the incident, injury, and the extent of any loss of consciousness may be useful in later assessment as well as in the preparation of subsequent medicolegal reports.

Many people attend hospital emergency departments for minor cuts, bruises, or pain, or for "a check up" after being involved in an incident, whereas others attend their general practitioner. Immediate distress is common. Clear explanation, advice, and discussion at the outset can prevent later problems in returning to normal activities and enable early recognition of psychological and social consequences. A sympathetic approach is needed that includes suitable analgesia, reassurance about the likely resolution of symptoms, and encouragement to return to normal activity. Some patients may already be considering compensation, and records should be kept with this in mind.

Advice about return to work and other activities
Patients with painful injuries that should improve within days or weeks are often uncertain how to behave and how soon to return to work. The assessment is an opportunity to give advice about this. Patients need information on the cause of their symptoms, their likely impact on daily life, and a positive plan for return to normal activity; this includes discussing the type of work normally done, the employer's attitude to time away from work, and opportunities for a graded increase in activity. Good, rapid communication between hospital and primary care is essential.

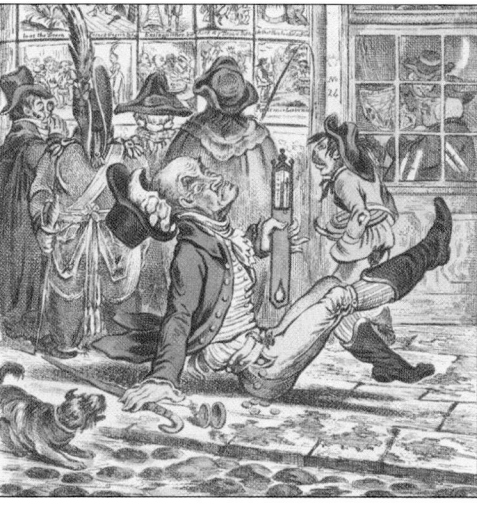

Detail of *Very Slippy Weather* by James Gillray (1757-1815)

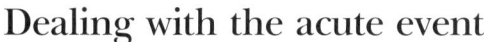

Lifetime prevalence of specific traumatic events (n=2181)

Type of trauma	Prevalence
Assault	38%
Serious car or motor vehicle crash	28%
Other serious accident or injury	14%
Fire, flood, earthquake, or other natural disaster	17%
Other shocking experience	43%
Diagnosed with a life threatening illness	5%
Learning about traumas to others	62%
Sudden, unexpected death of close friend or relative	60%
Any trauma	90%

Immediate effects of frightening trauma

- Causes a varied picture of anxiety, numbness, dissociation (feeling distanced from events, having fragmentary memories), and sometimes apparently inappropriate calmness
- Those who believe they are the innocent victims of others' misbehaviour are often angry, and this may be exacerbated by subsequent frustrations
- The term "acute stress disorder" is now used for a combination of distress, intrusive memories (flashbacks, nightmares), avoidance, and numbing in the months after the trauma. It occurs in 20-50% of those who have suffered major trauma
- The severity of emotional symptoms is much more closely related to how frightening the trauma was than to the severity of the injury; even uninjured victims may suffer considerable distress
- Severe distress is usually temporary but indicates a risk of long term post-traumatic symptoms

Immediate management

- Physical treatment, including adequate analgesia
- Sympathetic discussion of acute distress
- Explanation and appropriate reassurance about treatment and prognosis
- Appropriate encouragement for graded return to work and other activities
- Indicate what help will be available for continuing psychological symptoms and social problems
- Information and support to relatives

Immediate psychological interventions

Many employers and medical and voluntary groups recommend routine "debriefing" after frightening trauma. However, the evidence shows this is not only ineffective but may be harmful.

It is better, therefore, to concentrate on the immediate relief of distress through support and sympathetic reassurance and on practical help, while encouraging further early consultation if problems persist. This is especially so in groups who may be regularly exposed to frightening and distressing circumstances, such as members of the armed forces, police, and ambulance staff. Severe immediate distress and perception of the trauma as having been very frightening indicate an increased risk of chronic post-traumatic symptoms, and early review is recommended to identify those who need extra help. Victims of crime can be helped by referral to the charity Victim Support.

Later consequences and care

Treatment should include clear, agreed plans for mobilisation and return to optimal activity. Physiotherapists are often involved in rehabilitation and need to be aware of the psychological as well as the physical factors that are perpetuating disability. If necessary, a multidisciplinary approach should be established.

Chronic pain and disability

A small number of those who have suffered trauma continue to complain of physical symptoms and disabilities that are difficult to explain. Investigations are negative or ambiguous, and the relationship between doctors and patients may become fraught. Doctors may feel their patient is disabled for psychological reasons, whereas patients may feel that doctors do not believe that their symptoms are real and that they are unsympathetic and are not offering appropriate treatment.

Arguments about whether symptoms are physical or psychological are rarely helpful. Instead, it is essential to agree a coordinated behavioural and rehabilitative approach with patient and family that aims to achieve the maximum improvement. Unfortunately, there is a shortage of appropriate multidisciplinary specialist services for such people. This leaves primary care teams in the key role in monitoring progress and implementing a biopsychosocial approach to rehabilitation.

Psychological symptoms and syndromes

Depression, post-traumatic stress disorder, and phobic anxiety are common after frightening trauma and can be severe, whether or not there is evidence of previous psychological and social vulnerability. These psychological complications are not closely related to the severity of any physical injury. The general principles of assessment are those for similar psychological problems occurring in the absence of trauma.

Depression—A failure to recognise depression is distressingly common, perhaps because care focuses on physical injuries. Inquiries about depressive symptoms should therefore be routine.

Post-traumatic stress disorder is also common and disabling. It is characterised by intrusive memories of the trauma, avoidance of reminders of it, and chronic arousal and distress. It may be complicated by alcohol misuse. It usually has an early onset in the first few weeks (acute stress disorder). Many people improve rapidly but, if symptoms are still present two or three months after the injury, they are likely to persist for much longer. A few cases have a delayed onset. Psychological treatment is effective.

Phobic anxiety may be associated with post-traumatic stress disorder but can occur separately. A particularly common form

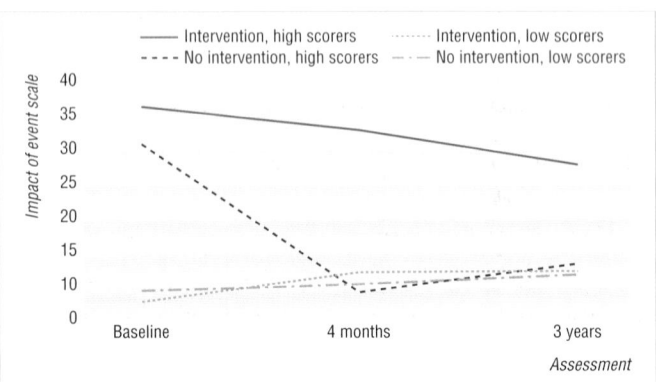

Effect of immediate debriefing on victims of road traffic injury. Those with high initial scores on the impact of events scale (intrusive thoughts and avoidance) had worse outcome than untreated controls at 4 months and 3 years

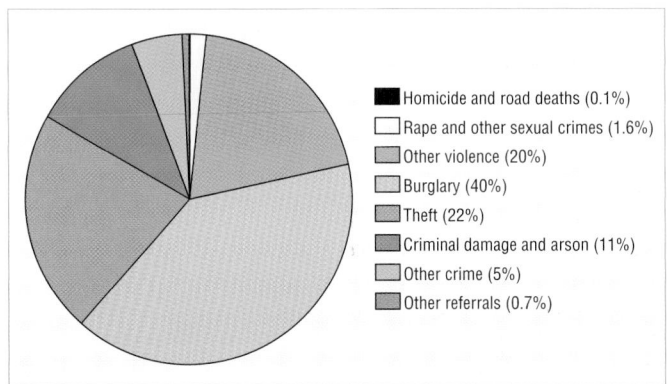

Reasons for people being offered help by Victim Support 1997-8

Unexplained and disproportionate disability and pain

- Lack of explanation or overcautious advice often leads to misunderstandings and secondary disability
- Delays in assessment and treatment exacerbate problems and make treatment more difficult
- Lack of coordination (between general practice, physiotherapy, hospital, etc) frequently exacerbates problems
- Low mood, misunderstandings, and inactivity worsen pain and disability
- Agree on consistent, collaborative plans with patient and family
- Early access to specialist rehabilitation and pain clinics providing high quality cognitive and behavioural psychological treatments

---

Psychologically determined consequences of trauma

- Acute anxiety, numbing, arousal (acute stress disorder)
- Anxiety disorder
- Major depressive disorder
- Post-traumatic symptoms and disorder
- Avoidance and phobic anxiety
- Pain and apparently disproportionate disability
- Unexplained physical symptoms
- Impact on family (such as family arguments, depression in family members)

Cognitive behavioural approach to treating post-traumatic stress disorder

- *Talking it through*—Encourage victim to discuss and relive feelings about the incident
- *Tackling avoidance*—Discuss graded increase in activities, such as return to travel after a road crash
- *Coping with anxiety*—Anxiety management techniques (relaxation, distraction)
- *Dealing with anger*—Encourage discussion of incident and of feelings
- *Overcoming sleep problems*—Emphasise importance of regular sleep habits and avoidance of excessive alcohol and caffeine
- *Treat associated depression*—Antidepressant drugs, limited role for hypnotics immediately after trauma

is anxiety about travel, both as a driver and as a passenger, after a road traffic crash. This anxiety may lead to distress and limitation of activities and lifestyle. Early advice about the use of anxiety management techniques and the need for a graded return to normal travel is helpful, but more specialist behavioural treatment may be required and is usually effective.

Detection of psychological problems
During a clinical assessment, a few brief screening questions can be useful as a guide to identify depression, anxiety, post-traumatic stress disorder and drinking problems. It is often helpful to speak to someone close to the victim who can offer an independent view.

Personal injury and compensation
Victims who believe that others are to blame for their trauma increasingly consult specialist lawyers, who are alert to psychiatric complications such as post-traumatic stress disorder and phobic avoidance. Acrimonious discussion about a small number of controversial cases of alleged exaggeration and simulation has obscured a more productive discussion of psychiatric disorder.

Head injury
Most head injuries are mild. These were once believed to be without consequences, but recent evidence has suggested that almost half of patients experiencing mild head injuries (Glasgow coma scale 13-15) remain appreciably disabled a year later. The effects of more severe head injuries on personality and cognitive performance may be greater than is apparent in a clinical interview and commonly affect "executive" functions such as social judgment and decision making.

Such deficits are often not detected by standard bedside screening tools such as the mini-mental state examination. Patients with head injury should therefore not be pushed to return to demanding activities too quickly, and there should be a low threshold for seeking a specialist opinion or undertaking psychometric assessment.

Consequences for others

Family members may also suffer distress, especially if they have been involved in the traumatic incident. Seeing the relatives of the traumatised person is usually helpful in the management of persistent problems.

Those involved in treating trauma will encounter particularly distressing incidents with severely injured victims and distraught relatives. These often occur when those involved in treatment are working under considerable pressure. Clear procedures for training and support of staff are essential. For those working in large emergency services the provision of regular specialist support is advisable.

Types of trauma

The pattern of consequences varies with the type of trauma experienced. All services that see trauma emergencies need management plans for psychological as well as medical care. This includes planning for major events in which there are many victims and for the much commoner road traffic and other incidents in which there are often several victims, some of whom may be severely injured and who may well be related or know one another. Emergency departments and primary care need procedures for helping the patients and for supporting the staff that are involved.

Treating avoidance and phobic anxiety
- *Diary keeping*–Encourage detailed diary of activity and associated problems as a basis for planning and monitoring progress
- *Anxiety (stress) management*–Relaxation, distraction, and cognitive procedure for use in stressful situations
- *Graded practice*–Discuss a hierarchy of increasing activities; emphasise importance of not being overambitious and need to be consistent in following step by step plan

---

Compensation
- Simulation of disability and exaggeration are uncommon in routine clinical contacts
- Many victims want recognition of their suffering as much as financial compensation
- Innocent victims of trauma are generally slower to return to work than those victims who accept that they were to blame
- Financial and social consequences of trauma and blighting of ambitions may be considerable and are often unrecognised
- Compensation procedures and reports may hinder development and agreement about treatment and active rehabilitation
- Compensation may allow interim payments and funding of specialist care to treat complications and prevent chronic disability

---

Head injury
- Assessment should involve questions about possible unconsciousness and post-traumatic amnesia
- Cognitive consequences of minor head injury are often not recognised
- Minor impairments may be obscured in clinical situations but be disabling in work and everyday activities
- Recovery may be prolonged
- Complaints of confusion and poor memory can be due to depression
- Specialist assessment may be needed

Relatives' needs
Immediately after severe or frightening trauma
- Make comfortable
- Inform relatives of trauma in a sympathetic manner
- Practical assistance
- Clear information

Later
- Information about injuries, treatment, and prognosis
- Discuss effects on everyday life
- Discuss needs for practical help and availability
- Ask about possible psychiatric problems and indicate help available

---

Types of trauma
- *Occupational*–Return to work often slower than in other types of injury. Liaison with employer essential. Compensation issues may impede return to work
- *Sporting*–May be associated with physical unfitness or with inappropriate activity for age
- *Domestic*–Assess role of alcohol, consider possible family and other problems, assess risk of further incidents
- *Assault (including sexual)*–Assess role of alcohol, keep detailed records, suggest availability of help for major, and especially for sexual, assault
- *Road traffic crash*–Psychological complications may occur even if no significant physical injury. Whiplash injuries should be treated by well planned mobilisation and encouragement, together with alertness to possible psychological complications

Disasters

All medical services and other institutions should have a disaster plan that is readily available and regularly reviewed. It should include a specification for immediate psychological care and information, together with proactive follow up so that psychological problems are identified early. Those involved in coping with disasters also require support and encouragement, and a minority may require specialist psychological help. The disaster plan should also set out procedures for giving information to relatives and offering them practical help.

Conclusion

The psychological aspects of trauma may be important, even when injury seems trivial. Clear, sympathetic care, which takes account of patients' needs, can do much to promote optimal recovery. Specialist advice should be sought for persistent problems within the first few months of an injury. Long delays in providing adequate assessment and treatment lead to unnecessary suffering and disability and may make such problems much more difficult to treat.

The print *Very Slippy Weather* is reproduced with permission of Leeds Museum and Art Galleries and Bridgeman Art Library. The table of lifetime prevalence of traumatic events is adapted from Breslau et al. *Arch Gen Psychiatry* 1998;55:626-32. The graph of effect of immediate debriefing on the psychiatric wellbeing of victims of road traffic injury is adapted from Mayou et al *Br J Psychiatry* 2000;176:590-4. The figure showing reasons for people being offered help by Victim Support is adapted from *Information in the Criminal Justice System in England and Wales. Digest 4*, London: Home Office, 1999.

Evidence based summary

- Cognitive behaviour therapy is effective in treating post-traumatic stress disorder
- Early critical incident debriefing after trauma is potentially harmful

Sherman JJ. Effects of psychotherapeutic treatments for PTSD: a meta-analysis of controlled clinical trials. *J Trauma Stress* 1998;11:413-36

Wessely S, Rose S, Bisson J. Brief psychological interventions ("debriefing") for trauma-related symptoms and the prevention of post traumatic stress disorder *Cochrane Database Syst Rev* 2999;(2):CD00050

Suggested reading

- Mayou RA, Bryant B. Outcome in consecutive emergency department attenders following a road traffic accident. *Br J Psychiatry* 2001;179:528-34
- McDonald AS, Davey GCL. Psychiatric disorders and accidental injury. *Clin Psychol Rev* 1996;16:105
- NIH Consensus Development Panel on Rehabilitation of Persons with Traumatic Brain Injury. Rehabilitation of persons with traumatic brain injury. *JAMA* 1999;282:974-83

---

10 Fatigue

Michael Sharpe, David Wilks

Fatigue can refer to a subjective symptom of malaise and aversion to activity or to objectively impaired performance. It has both physical and mental aspects. The symptom of fatigue is a poorly defined feeling, and careful inquiry is needed to clarify complaints of "fatigue," "tiredness," or "exhaustion" and to distinguish lack of energy from loss of motivation or sleepiness, which may be pointers to specific diagnoses (see below).

Prevalence—Like blood pressure, subjective fatigue is normally distributed in the population. The prevalence of continuously significant fatigue depends on the threshold chosen for severity (usually defined in terms of associated disability) and persistence. Surveys report that 5-20% of the general population suffer from such persistent and troublesome fatigue. Fatigue is twice as common in women as in men but is not strongly associated with age or occupation. It is one of the commonest presenting symptoms in primary care, being the main complaint of 5-10% of patients and an important subsidiary symptom in a further 5-10%.

Fatigue as a symptom—Patients generally regard fatigue as important (because it is disabling), whereas doctors do not (because it is diagnostically non-specific). This discrepancy is a potent source of potential difficulty in the doctor-patient relationship. Fatigue may present in association with established medical and psychiatric conditions or be idiopathic. Irrespective of cause, it has a major impact on day to day functioning and quality of life. Without treatment, the prognosis of patients with idiopathic fatigue is surprisingly poor; half those seen in general practice with fatigue are still fatigued six months later.

Causes of fatigue

The physiological and psychological mechanisms underlying subjective fatigue are poorly understood. Fatigue may rather be usefully regarded as a final common pathway for a variety of causal factors. These can be split into predisposing, precipitating, and perpetuating factors.

Predisposing factors include being female and a history of either fatigue or depression.

Precipitating factors include acute physical stresses such as infection with Epstein-Barr virus, psychological stresses such as bereavement, and social stresses such as work problems.

Perpetuating factors include physical inactivity, emotional disorders, ongoing psychological or social stresses, and abnormalities of sleep. These factors should be sought as part of the clinical assessment.

Other physiological factors such as immunological abnormalities and slightly low cortisol concentration are of research interest but not clinical value.

Diagnoses associated with fatigue

Among patients who present with severe chronic fatigue as their main complaint, only a small proportion will be suffering from a recognised medical disease. In no more than 10% of patients presenting with fatigue in primary care is a disease cause found. The rate is even lower in patients seen in secondary care.

Fatigue is a major symptom of many psychiatric disorders, but for a substantial proportion of patients with fatigue the

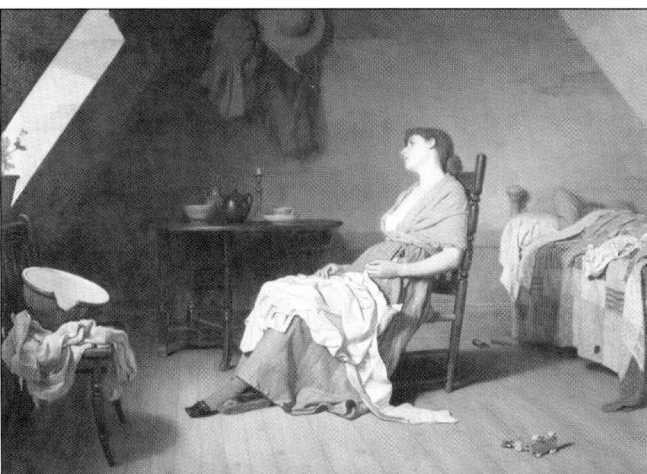

Weary 1887 by Edward Radford (1831-1920)

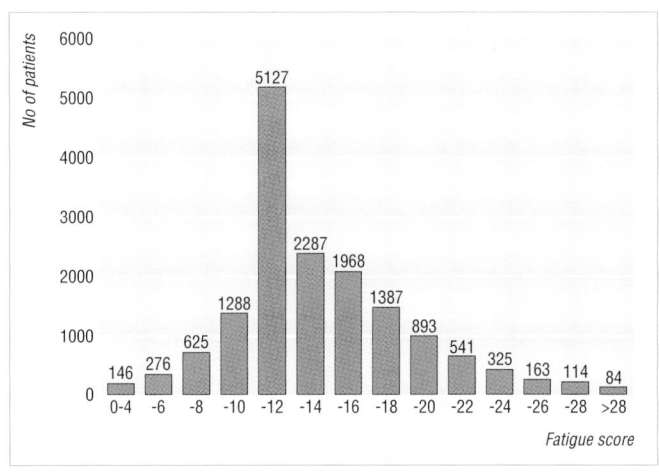

Distribution of the complaint of fatigue in the population

Medical conditions that may present with apparently unexplained fatigue

- *General*—Anaemia, chronic infection, autoimmune disease, cancer
- *Endocrine disease*—Diabetes, hypothyroidism, hypoadrenalism
- *Sleep disorders*—Obstructive sleep apnoea and other sleep disorders
- *Neuromuscular*—Myositis, multiple sclerosis
- *Gastrointestinal*—Liver disease
- *Cardiovascular*—Chronic heart disease
- *Respiratory*—Chronic lung disease

---

symptom remains unexplained or idiopathic. In general, the more severe the fatigue and the larger the number of associated somatic (and unexplained) complaints, then the greater the disability and the greater the likelihood of a diagnosis of depression.

Chronic fatigue syndromes

Chronic fatigue syndrome is a useful descriptive term for prominent physical and mental fatigue with muscular pain and other symptoms. It overlaps with another descriptive term, fibromyalgia, that has often been used when muscle pain is predominant but in which fatigue is almost universal. There is also substantial overlap of the diagnoses with other symptom based syndromes, the so called functional somatic syndromes.

The term myalgic encephalomyelitis (or encephalopathy) has been used in Britain and elsewhere to describe a poorly understood illness in which a prominent symptom is chronic fatigue exacerbated by activity. This is a controversial diagnosis that some regard as simply another name for chronic fatigue syndrome and that others regard as a distinct condition. This article will focus on chronic fatigue syndrome.

Prevalence and outcome—Chronic fatigue syndrome can be diagnosed in up to 2% of primary care patients. Untreated, the prognosis is poor, with only about 10% of patients recovering in a two to four years. A preoccupation with medical causes seems to be a negative prognostic factor.

Assessment and formulation

History—The nature of the fatigue is an important clue to diagnosis, and it is therefore important to clarify patients' complaints. Fatigue described as loss of interest and enjoyment (anhedonia) points to depression. Prominent sleepiness suggests a sleep disorder. The history should also cover
- Systematic inquiry for diseases and medications often associated with fatigue
- Symptoms of depression anxiety and sleep disorder
- Patients' own understanding of their illness and how they cope with it
- Current social stresses.

Examination—Both a physical and mental state examination must be performed in every case, to seek medical and psychiatric diagnoses associated with fatigue.

Routine investigations—If there are no specific indications for special investigations, a standard set of screening tests is adequate.

Special investigations—Immunological and virological tests are generally unhelpful as routine investigations. Sleep studies can be useful in excluding other diagnoses, especially obstructive sleep apnoea and narcolepsy.

Psychological assessment—It is important to inquire fully about patients' understanding of their illness (questions may include "What do you think is wrong with you?" and "What do you think the cause is?"). Patients may be worried that the fatigue is a symptom of a severe, as yet undiagnosed, disease or that activity will cause a long term worsening of their condition.

Formulation—A formulation that distinguishes predisposing, precipitating, and multiple perpetuating factors is valuable in providing an explanation to patients and for targeting intervention.

General management

Persistent fatigue requires active management, preferably before it has become chronic. When a specific disease cause of fatigue

---

Psychiatric diagnoses commonly associated with fatigue
- Depression
- Anxiety and panic
- Eating disorders
- Substance misuse disorders
- Somatisation disorder

Diagnostic criteria for chronic fatigue syndrome

Inclusion criteria
- Clinically evaluated, medically unexplained fatigue of at least 6 months' duration that is
  Of new onset (not life long)
  Not result of ongoing exertion
  Not substantially alleviated by rest
  Associated with a substantial reduction in previous level of activities
- Occurrence of 4 or more of the following symptoms
  Subjective memory impairment, sore throat, tender lymph nodes, muscle pain, joint pain, headache, unrefreshing sleep, post-exertional malaise lasting more than 24 hours

Exclusion criteria
- Active, unresolved, or suspected medical disease or psychotic, melancholic, or bipolar depression (but not uncomplicated major depression), psychotic disorders, dementia, anorexia or bulimia nervosa, alcohol or other substance misuse, severe obesity

---

Screening tests for fatigue
- Full blood count
- Erythrocyte sedimentation rate or C reactive protein
- Liver function tests
- Urea, electrolytes, and calcium
- Thyroid stimulating hormone and thyroid function tests
- Creatine kinase
- Urine and blood tests for glucose
- Urine test for protein

Factors to consider in a formulation of chronic fatigue

	Predisposing cause	Precipitating cause	Perpetuating cause
Biological	Biological vulnerability	Acute disease	Pathophysiology Excessive inactivity Sleep disorder Side effects of drug treatment Untreated disease
Psychological	Vulnerable personality	Stress	Depression Unhelpful beliefs about cause Fearful avoidance of activity
Social	Lack of support	Life events Social or work stress	Reinforcement of unhelpful beliefs Social or work stress

can be identified this should be treated. If no disease diagnosis can be made, or if medical treatment of disease fails to relieve the fatigue, a broader biopsychosocial management strategy is required. A discussion with the patient about fatigue and its treatment can be supplemented with written material (see below).

Patients should be told that they are suffering from a common and treatable condition that the doctor takes seriously and for which behavioural treatment can be helpful. While patients may be concerned about possible disease and the need for medical investigation and treatment, it can be explained that no disease has been found, and hence there is no disease based treatment, but that with help there is a great deal that the patients can do themselves.

Identifying unhelpful beliefs—Potentially unhelpful beliefs should be discussed. If a patient has a simple aetiological model (such as "It is all due to a virus") an alternative approach based on a biopsychosocial formulation can be outlined. This has the advantage of highlighting potential perpetuating factors, as these may be regarded as obstacles to recovery. Doctor and patient can then work together to overcome these. It is rarely productive to argue over the best name for the illness; instead, the emphasis should be on agreeing a positive and open minded approach to rehabilitation.

Managing activity and avoidance—Gradual increases in activity can be advised unless there is a clear contraindication. It is critical, however, to distinguish between carefully graded increases carried out in collaboration with patients and "forced" exercise. It is also important to explain that erratic variation between overactivity on "good" days and subsequent collapse does not help long term recovery and that "stabilising" activity is a prerequisite to graded increases.

Depression and anxiety—If there is evidence of depression a trial of an antidepressant drug is worth while. Patients with fatigue are often sensitive to the side effects of antidepressants. However, if they are given adequate information about what to expect when treatment begins, with small doses, most patients can tolerate them. Randomised trials have shown psychological therapies such as cognitive behaviour therapy to be equally effective for mild to moderate depression.

Managing occupational and social stresses—Patients who remain in work may be overstressed by it. Those who have left work may be inactive and demoralised and may not wish to return to the same job. These situations require a problem solving approach to consider how to manage work demands, achieve a return to work, or to plan an alternative career.

Drug Treatments for Fatigue—A variety of pharmacological drugs including stimulants and steroids have been advocated for the treatment of fatigue. There is a limited evidence base for any of these pharmacological treatments, most of which may lead to substantial adverse effects. The role for these drugs is therefore limited and they should only be prescribed with great caution.

Referral for specialist management

Most patients with fatigue are managed in primary care, but certain groups may require referral to specialist care:
- Children with chronic fatigue
- Patients in whom the general practitioner suspects occult disease
- Patients with severe psychiatric illness
- Patients requiring specialist management of sleep disorders
- Patients unresponsive to management in primary care.

Management of chronic fatigue

1 Assessment
 Empathise
 History
 Examination
 Limited investigation
 Biopsychosocial formulations
2 Treat treatable medical and psychiatric conditions
3 Help patient to overcome perpetuating factors
 Educate
 Reduce distress
 Gradual increase in activity
 Solve social and occupational problems
4 Follow up

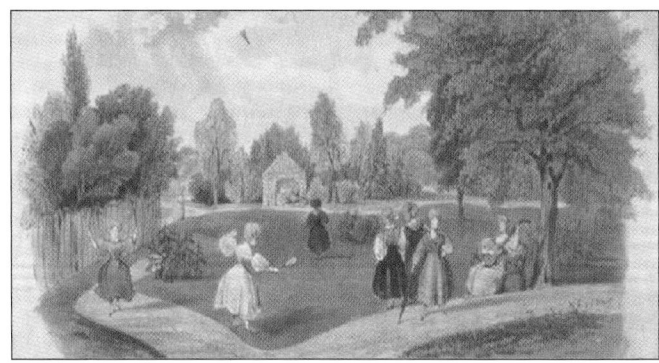

Patients should be encouraged to gradually increase their activity ("Mrs Bradbury's establishment for the recovery of ladies nervously affected")

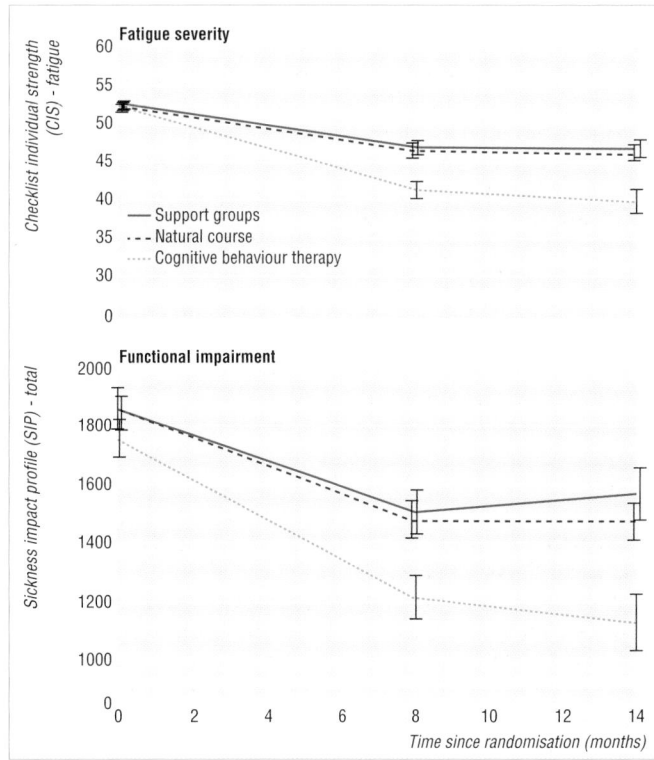

Efficacy of cognitive behaviour therapy for treating chronic fatigue syndrome

---

What is cognitive behaviour therapy?

- Brief pragmatic psychological therapy
- Targets beliefs and behaviours that might perpetuate symptoms
- An established treatment for depression and anxiety
- Has been adapted for somatic complaints of pain and fatigue
- Requires a skilled therapist

Referral may be to a physician or psychiatrist as is deemed most appropriate. Psychologists may be able to offer cognitive behaviour therapy. Where available, joint medical and psychiatric clinics are ideally suited to the assessment of chronic fatigue and related problems. It is essential there is close liaison between primary and specialist care to ensure a clear, consistent, and encouraging approach by all concerned.

Rehabilitation

Rehabilitation based on behavioural principles is currently the most effective specialist treatment approach.

Cognitive behaviour therapy is a collaborative psychological rehabilitation that incorporates graded increases in activity but also pays greater attention to patients' beliefs and concerns.

Graded exercise therapy is a structured progressive exercise programme administered and carefully monitored by a therapist.

Both may be used in conjunction with antidepressant drugs. Both have been found to be effective in randomised trials of hospital referred cases of chronic fatigue syndrome. Some general practitioners are able to provide graded exercise or cognitive behaviour therapy in their practice or clinic. Others may wish to refer to a trained therapist.

Conclusion

Fatigue is a ubiquitous symptom that is important to patients and has a major impact on their quality of life. It remains poorly understood and has hitherto probably been not been given adequate attention by doctors. Early and active management of fatigue in primary care may prevent progression to chronicity. Patients who have developed a chronic fatigue syndrome can benefit from specific treatments. Paying more attention to the symptom of fatigue may help to avoid the distress and poor outcome that is associated with patients feeling that their problems are neither accepted nor understood. It may also reduce the numbers who turn to a variety of unproved, and even harmful, alternative approaches.

What is graded exercise therapy?

- Explanation of fatigue as a physiological consequence of inactivity, poor sleep, and disturbed circadian rhythms
- Discussion, agreement, and implementation of graded exercise plans
- Monitoring of progress and setting of appropriate new targets

---

Evidence based summary

- Chronic fatigue syndrome is a descriptive term for a disabling syndrome that probably has multiple causes (physical and psychological)
- Graded exercise and cognitive behaviour therapies are effective in treating chronic fatigue syndrome

Wessely S. Chronic fatigue: symptom and syndrome. *Ann Intern Med* 2001;134:838-43

Whiting P, Bagnall AM, Sowden AJ, Cornell JE, Mulrow CD, Ramirez G. Interventions for the treatment and management of chronic fatigue syndrome: a systematic review. *JAMA* 2001;286:1360-8

Further reading

- Wessely S, Hotopf M, Sharpe M. *Chronic fatigue and its syndromes.* Oxford: Oxford University Press, 1998
- Campling F, Sharpe M. *Chronic fatigue syndrome: the facts.* Oxford: Oxford University Press, 2000
- Reid S, Chalder T, Cleare A, Hotopf M, Wessely S. Chronic fatigue syndrome. *Clinical Evidence* 2001 (Nov)

The painting *Weary* is held at Russell-Cotes Art Gallery and Museum, Bournemouth, and is reproduced with permission of Bridgeman Art Library. The graph of distribution of fatigue in the population is adapted from Pawlikowska T, et al *BMJ* 1994;308:763-6. The box of diagnostic criteria for chronic fatigue syndrome is adapted from Fukuda K, et al *Ann Intern Med* 1994;121:953-9. The print of "Mrs Bradbury's establishment for the recovery of ladies nervously affected" is reproduced with permission of Wellcome Library. The graph showing efficacy of cognitive behaviour therapy is adapted from Prins JB, et al *Lancet* 2001;357:841-7.

11 Musculoskeletal pain

Chris J Main, Amanda C de C Williams

Musculoskeletal symptoms of various types (neck pain, limb pain, low back pain, joint pain, chronic widespread pain) are a major reason for consultation in primary care. This article uses the example of low back pain because it is particularly common and there is a substantial evidence base for its management. The principles of management outlined are also applicable to non-specific musculoskeletal symptoms in general.

The increasing prevalence of musculoskeletal pain, including back pain, has been described as an epidemic. Pain complaints are usually self limiting, but if they become chronic the consequences are serious. These include the distress of patients and their families and consequences for employers in terms of sickness absence and for society as a whole in terms of welfare benefits and lost productivity. Many causes for musculoskeletal pain have been identified. Psychological and social factors have been shown to play a major role in exacerbating the biological substrate of pain by influencing pain perception and the development of chronic disability. This new understanding has led to a "biopsychosocial" model of back pain.

Research has also shown that there are many different reasons for patients to consult their doctor with pain—seeking cure or symptomatic relief, diagnostic clarification, reassurance, "legitimisation" of symptoms, or medical certification for work absence or to express distress, frustration, or anger. Doctors need to clarify which of these reasons apply to an individual and to respond appropriately.

Managing acute back pain

Most patients can be effectively managed with a combination of brief assessment and giving information, advice, analgesia, and appropriate reassurance. Minimal rest and an early return to work should be encouraged. Explanation and advice can be usefully supplemented with written material.

Doctors' tasks include not only the traditional provision of diagnosis, investigation, prescriptions, and sickness certificates but also giving accurate advice, information, and reassurance. Primary care and emergency department doctors are potentially powerful therapeutic agents and can provide effective immediate care, but they may also unintentionally promote progression to chronic pain. The risk of chronicity is reduced by

- Paying attention to the psychological aspects of symptom presentation
- Avoiding unnecessary, excessive, or inappropriate investigation
- Avoiding inconsistent care (which may cause patients to become overcautious)
- Giving advice on preventing recurrence (such as by sensible lifting and avoiding excessive loads).

Research evidence supports a change of emphasis from treating symptoms to early prevention of factors that result in progression to chronicity. This has led to the development of new back pain management guidelines for both medical management and occupational health. The shift in emphasis from rest and immobilisation to active self management requires broadening the focus of the consultation from examination of symptoms alone to assessment, which includes

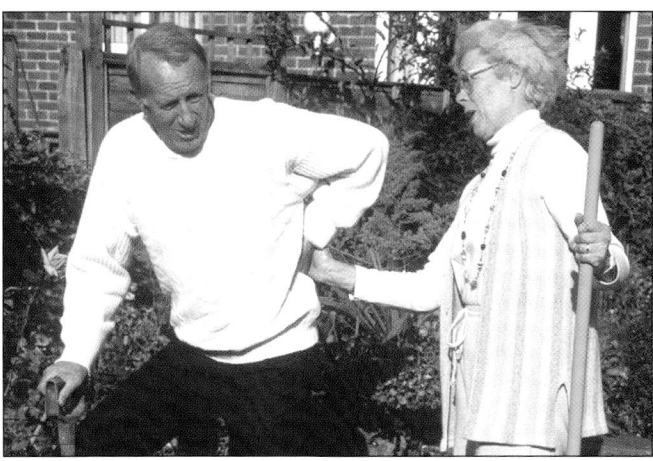

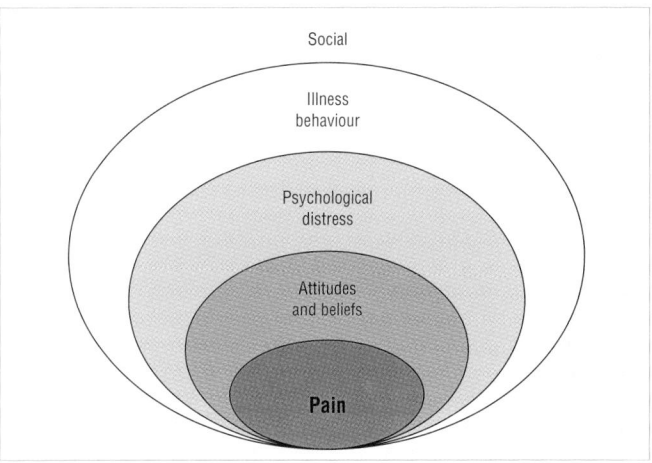

Biopsychosocial model of the clinical presentation and assessment of low back pain and disability at a point in time

---

Excerpt from information booklet *The Back Book**

It's your back

Backache is not a serious disease and it should not cripple you unless you let it. We have tried to show you the best way to deal with it. The important thing now is for you to get on with your life. How your backache affects you depends on how you react to the pain and what you do about it yourself.

There is no instant answer. You will have your ups and downs for a while—that is normal. But look at it this way

There are two types of sufferer

One who avoids activity, and one who copes

- The *avoider* gets frightened by the pain and worries about the future
- The *avoider* is afraid that hurting always means further damage—it doesn't
- The *avoider* rests a lot and waits for the pain to get better
- The *coper* knows that the pain will get better and does not fear the future
- The *coper* carries on as normally as possible
- The *coper* deals with the pain by being positive, staying active, or staying at work

*Roland M et al, Stationery Office, 2002.

patients' understanding of their pain and how they behave in response to it. The shift towards self directed pain management recasts the role of primary care doctor to the more rewarding one of guide or coach rather than a mere "mechanic."

Identify risk factors for chronicity

Guidelines for primary care management of acute back pain highlight the identification of risk factors for chronicity. A useful approach has been developed in New Zealand. It aims to involve all interested parties—patient, the patient's family, healthcare professionals, and, importantly, the patient's employer. Four groups of risk factors or "flags" for chronicity are accompanied by recommended assessment strategies, which include the use of screening questionnaires, a set of structured interview prompts, and a guide to behavioural management. The focus is on key psychological factors or "yellow flags" that favour chronicity:

- The belief that back pain is due to progressive pathology
- The belief that back pain is harmful or severely disabling
- The belief that avoidance of activity will help recovery
- A tendency to low mood and withdrawal from social interaction
- The expectation that passive treatments rather than active self management will help.

The assessment of "red flags" will identify the small number of patients who need referral for an urgent surgical opinion. Similarly, patients with declared suicidal intent require immediate psychiatric referral. These two groups of patients need to be managed separately.

For the vast majority of patients, however, the identification of contributory psychological and social factors should be seen as an investigation of the normal range of reactions to pain rather than the seeking of psychopathology. Questions in the form of interview prompts have been designed to elicit potential psychosocial barriers to recovery in the "yellow flags" system. They can be used at the time of initial presentation by the general practitioner.

Establish collaboration

Recent studies of miscommunications between doctors and patients with pain show that adequate assessment and collaborative management cannot be achieved without good communication between doctors and patients: only then will patients fully disclose their concerns.

The essence of good communication is to work toward understanding a patient's problem from his or her own perspective. In order to do this, the doctor must first gain the patient's confidence. A patient who has been convinced that the doctor takes the pain seriously will give credence to what the doctor says. Unfortunately, the converse is more common, and patients who feel that a doctor has dismissed or under-rated their pain are unlikely to reveal key information or to adhere to treatment advice.

Enhance accurate beliefs and self management strategies

It is easy to overlook the value of simple measures. Many patients respond positively to clear and simple advice, which enables them to manage and control their own symptoms.

Factors associated with chronicity and outcome

Distress
- Symptom awareness and concern
- Depressive reactions; helplessness

Beliefs about pain and disability
- Significance and controllability
- Fears and misunderstandings about pain

Behavioural factors
- Guarded movements and avoidance patterns
- Coping style and strategies

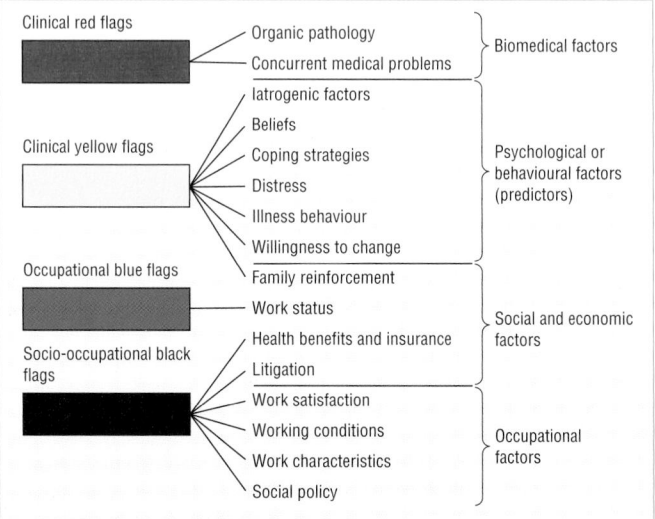

The clinical flags approach to obstacles to recovery from back pain and aspects of assessment

Structured interview prompts

- What do you understand is the cause of your back pain?
- What are you expecting will help you?
- How are others responding to your back pain (employer, coworkers, and family)?
- What are you doing to cope with back pain?
- Have you had time off work in the past with back pain?
- Do you think that you will ever return to work? When?

Guidelines for collaborative management of patients with pain

- Listen carefully to the patient
- Carefully observe the patient's behaviour
- Attend not only to what is said but also how it is said
- Attempt to understand how the patient feels
- Offer encouragement to disclose fears and feelings
- Offer reassurance that you accept the reality of the pain
- Correct misunderstandings or miscommunications about the consultation
- Offer appropriate challenges to unhelpful thoughts and biases (such as catastrophising)
- Understand the patient's general social and economic circumstances

Examples of simple management strategies

- Explain the difference between "hurt" and "harm"
- Reassure patients about the future and the benign nature of their symptoms
- Help patients regain control over pain
- Get patients to "pace" activities—that is, perform activities in manageable, graded stages
- Advise that analgesic drugs be taken on a regular rather than a pain contingent basis
- Set realistic goals such as small increases in activity
- Suggest rewards for successful achievement (such as listening to some favourite music)

Some of these strategies may seem self evident or even trivial, but they are not. Only by building confidence slowly is it possible to prevent the development of invalidity. Occasionally patients will seem to "get stuck" and become demoralised or distressed. Suggesting ways to enhance positive self management can help maintain progress towards a more satisfactory lifestyle.

The success of the cognitive and behavioural approach described below has stimulated the development of secondary prevention programmes designed to prevent those with low back pain from becoming chronically incapacitated by it. Intervention programmes based on cognitive behaviour therapy have also been shown to be effective in reducing disability.

Manage distress and anger

If patients show evidence of distress or anger, find out why. Various strategies for dealing with distress and anger have been developed.

Managing disabling chronic back pain

A minority of patients become increasingly incapacitated and require more detailed management of what has become a chronic pain problem. Research has shown that the most important influences on the development of chronicity are psychological rather than biomechanical. The psychological factors are high levels of distress, misunderstandings about pain and its implications, and avoidance of activities associated with a fear of making pain worse.

For patients with established chronic disabling pain specialist referral is required. The treatment of choice is an interdisciplinary pain management programme (IPMP). In these programmes the focus is changed from pain to function, with particular emphasis on perceived obstacles to recovery.

These pain management programmes address the clinical flags. The most commonly used therapeutic approach is a cognitive-behavioural perspective with emphasis on self management. Treatment approaches based on cognitive and behavioural principles have been found to be more effective than traditional biomedical or biomechanically oriented interventions.

Specific chronic pain syndromes

Many specific and more widespread pain syndromes have been described—such as "chronic pain," late whiplash syndrome, chronic widespread pain, fibromyalgia, somatoform pain disorder, repetitive strain disorder. It seems unlikely that these are distinct entities, and they are best seen as overlapping descriptive terms that do not have specific aetiological significance. Multidisciplinary treatment that includes psychological, behavioural, and psychiatric assessment and interventions is usually required.

Conclusion

There needs to be a revolution in the day to day management of musculoskeletal pain. Not only do we need to abandon prolonged rest and enforced inactivity as a form of treatment, but we also need to appreciate that addressing patients' beliefs, distress, and coping strategies must be an integral part of management if it is to be effective.

Ways of enhancing positive self management

Get patients to
- Identify when they are thinking in unrealistic, unhelpful ways about their pain (such as "It will keep getting worse") and to change to making a more balanced positive evaluation
- Notice when they are becoming tense or angry and then take steps to interrupt their thoughts and to use relaxation strategies
- Change how they respond when the pain gets bad (such as pause and take a break)
- Document their progress
- Elicit and use the help of others to establish and maintain successful coping strategies

---

Key strategies for assessing and managing distress and anger associated with pain

- Distinguish distress associated with pain and disability from more general distress
- Identify iatrogenic misunderstandings
- Identify mistaken beliefs and fears
- Try to correct misunderstandings
- Identify iatrogenic distress and anger
- Listen and empathise
- Above all, don't get angry yourself

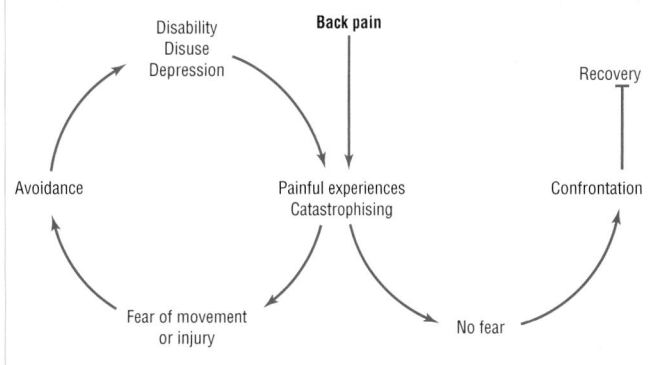

Effects of confrontation or avoidance of pain on outcome of episode of low back pain: fear of movement and re-injury can determine how some people recover from back pain while others develop chronic pain and disability

---

Defining characteristics of modern pain management programmes

- Focus on function rather than disease
- Focus on management rather than cure
- Integration of specific therapeutic ingredients
- Multidisciplinary management
- Emphasis on active rather than passive methods
- Emphasis on self care rather than simply receiving treatment

Lessons learnt in the management of chronic low back pain have direct relevance to the early and specialist management of musculoskeletal pain in general.

The photograph of a man with back pain is reproduced with permission of John Powell/Rex. The figure showing the biopsychosocial model of low back pain is adapted from Waddell G, *The back pain revolution*, Edinburgh: Churchill Livingstone, 1998. The figure showing the clinical flags approach to assessing back pain and the box of defining characteristics of modern pain management programmes are adapted from Main CJ and Spanswick CC, *Pain management: an interdisciplinary approach*, Edinburgh: Churchill-Livingstone, 2000. The boxes of guidelines for collaborative management of patients with pain, of key strategies for managing distress and anger associated with pain, of structured interview prompts, and of ways to enhance positive self management are adapted from Main CJ and Watson PJ, in Gifford L, ed, *Topical issues in pain*, vol 3, Falmouth: CNS Press (in press). The figure showing effects of confrontation or avoidance of pain on outcome of episode of low back pain is adapted from Vlaeyen JWS et al, *J Occup Rehabil* 1995;5:235-52.

Evidence based summary

- Acute back pain is best treated with minimal rest and rapid return to work and normal activity
- Psychological and behavioural responses to pain and social factors are the main determinants of chronic pain disability
- Specialist psychological treatments and pain management programmes are effective in treating chronic pain

Burton AK, Waddell G, Tillotson KM, Summerton N. Information and advice to patients with back pain can have a positive effect. A randomised controlled trial of a novel educational booklet in primary care. *Spine* 1999;24:2484-91

Linton SJ. A Review of psychological risk factors in back and neck pain. *Spine* 2000;25:1148-56

Morley SJ, Eccleston C, Williams A. Systematic review and meta-analysis of randomised controlled trials of cognitive behaviour therapy and behaviour therapy for chronic pain in adults, excluding headache. *Pain* 1999;80:1-13

Further reading

- Clinical Standards Advisory Group. *Clinical Standards Advisory Group report on back pain*. London: HMSO, 1994
- Kendall NAS, Linton SJ, Main CJ. *Guide to assessing psychosocial yellow flags in acute low back pain: risk factors for long term disability and work loss*. Wellington, NZ: Accident Rehabilitation and Compensation Insurance Corporation of New Zealand and the National Health Committee, 1997
- Royal College of General Practitioners. *Clinical guidelines for the management of acute low back pain*. London: RCGP, 1996
- Waddell G, Burton K. *Occupational health guidelines for the management of low back pain at work—evidence review*. London: Faculty of Occupational Medicine, 2000
- Roland M, Waddell G, Klaber-Moffett J, Burton AK, Main CJ. *The back book*. 2nd ed. Norwich: Stationery Office, 2002

12 Abdominal pain and functional gastrointestinal disorders

Elspeth Guthrie, David Thompson

Various functional gastrointestinal pain syndromes have been defined, but there is substantial overlap between them. There is also substantial overlap with other functional disorders such as chronic fatigue syndrome, fibromyalgia, and chronic pelvic pain. The classification system for functional gastrointestinal disorders (FGID) therefore remains controversial and is seldom used outside specialist and research settings. Furthermore, the psychological management of these different syndromes is essentially similar.

In primary care about half of the patients seen with gut complaints have FGID, the most common disorder being irritable bowel syndrome. A UK general practitioner is estimated to see eight patients with irritable bowel syndrome every week, one of whom will be presenting for the first time.

The quality of life of patients with chronic FGID is far poorer than in the general population, and is even significantly lower than in patients with many other chronic illnesses. These patients are not merely the "worried well." It is also important to resist the temptation to think of FGID as exclusively psychological disorders. A biopsychosocial approach is preferable. Physiological studies have suggested that patients with FGID have abnormal visceral sensation and abnormal patterns of bowel motility. Both psychological and physiological factors are involved, with the relative contribution of these varying among patients.

Aetiological factors include physiological and psychological predisposition, early life experience, and current social stresses. It has been shown that a combination of psychological factors and sensitisation of the gut after infection can trigger irritable bowel syndrome in adults.

Emotional distress—The degree of associated emotional distress with FGID depends on the treatment setting. In the community and general practice the prevalence of psychological distress in patients with functional abdominal pain is about 10-20%, whereas in clinic and outpatient settings it is 30-40%, and is even higher for patients who are "treatment resistant."

Abuse—Women with severe FGID often have a history of sexual and emotional abuse. This is as high as 30% in those attending gastroenterology clinics.

Initial management

Most patients with FGID have relatively mild symptoms and can be managed effectively in primary care. Only a third of patients seen in primary care with irritable bowel syndrome are referred to gastrointestinal specialists for further assessment and treatment.

Symptomatic treatment—Drug treatments for FGID are aimed at improving the predominant symptoms, such as constipation, diarrhoea, abdominal pain, or upper gastrointestinal symptoms. Standard treatments for lower bowel symptoms, depending on the predominant symptom, include dietary fibre, laxatives, antispasmodic agents (including anticholinergics and direct smooth muscle relaxants), and antidiarrhoeals. Treatment for upper gastrointestinal symptoms include H_2 receptor antagonists and prokinetics. There are several useful reviews of the efficacy of these agents in FGID (see further reading).

Functional gastrointestinal disorders

- Functional dyspepsia
- Ulcer-like dyspepsia
- Dysmotility-like dyspepsia
- Unspecified dyspepsia
- Functional diarrhoea
- Functional constipation

- Irritable bowel syndrome
- Functional abdominal bloating
- Unspecified functional bowel disorder
- Functional abdominal pain syndrome
- Unspecified functional abdominal pain

Diagnostic criteria for irritable bowel syndrome

In preceding 12 months at least 12 weeks of abdominal discomfort with 2 of 3 features: relieved with defecation, onset associated with change in frequency of stool, onset associated with change in form of stool
Supportive symptoms include

- Fewer than 3 bowel movements a week
- More than 3 bowel movements a day
- Straining during bowel movement
- Urgent bowel movements
- Feeling of incomplete bowel movement

- Hard or lumpy stools
- Loose or watery stools
- Passing mucus
- Abdominal fullness, bloating, or swelling

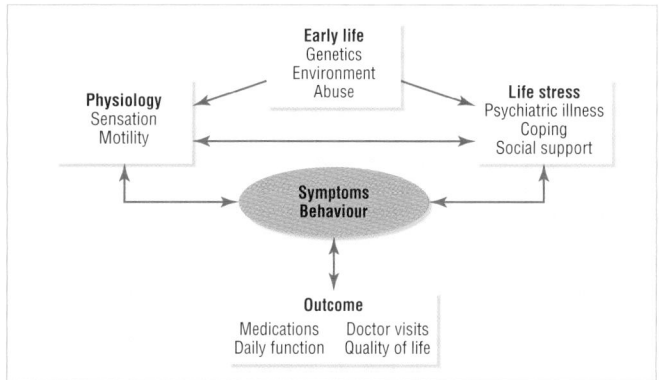

Biopsychosocial model for functional abdominal pain

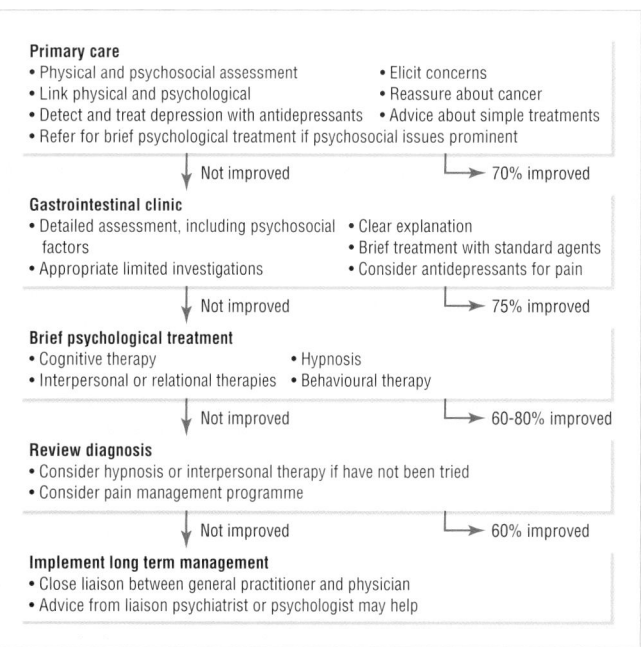

Algorithm for treating patients with functional gastrointestinal disorders

Psychological management—Initial management can be enhanced by incorporating brief psychological management strategies. Many patients with FGID are afraid that they have a serious underlying disease such as cancer, and attempts should be made to elicit such fears and address them. It is also important to provide a positive and credible explanation for the symptoms. The explanation should include both physiological and psychological factors. One way of explaining symptoms is to describe how the bowel is a segmented tube in which food is propelled down by the sequential squeezing of each segment. The nervous control of this system is delicate and complicated, and disruption of it consequently produces muscle spasm in the bowel wall, which results in pain and gas. Stress and other psychological factors such as anxiety cause bowel symptoms by affecting this nervous control.

Antidepressants—A recent meta-analysis of 12 randomised controlled trials of antidepressants for treating FGID concluded that they are moderately effective. On average, 3.2 patients need to be treated to substantially improve one patient's symptoms. Antidepressants should therefore be considered if there is clear evidence of a depressive disorder, but they may also help to reduce pain in the absence of depression.

Management of chronic problems

In the case of patients with chronic symptoms that have not responded to treatment, psychological factors are likely to be important. Doctors should try to elicit patients' concerns, seek evidence of emotional distress, and, over several consultations if necessary, help them to make tentative connections between psychological factors, life stresses, and the pain.

The following strategies are suggested:
- Set aside an appointment that is longer than usual, so there is time to deal with a patient's concerns. This is better than several fruitless, rushed consultations focusing only on symptoms
- Make sure that any investigations are based on the patient's history and examination. Do not allow yourself to be pushed into ordering investigations that are not clinically indicated. Try to avoid setting up a "referral matrix," with the patient being referred on from one specialty to another
- Emphasise the role that patients can play in improving or relieving pain by carrying out agreed strategies or exercises. Include the patient in decision about treatment options. Encourage membership of self help groups and organisations. The International Federation for Functional Gastrointestinal Disorders is a well respected organisation that provides useful information for patients. For patients with irritable bowel syndrome, the IBS Network is UK based and is also helpful
- Avoid changing treatments too often; improvement will be slow. Patients are likely to raise concerns about their condition at every consultation, so be prepared to give an explanation of the symptoms more than once. Make a note in the records of what you have said so that you don't contradict yourself
- Be prepared for patients to continually question your approach and think about ways to address this before each consultation. It may be helpful to discuss your management with a psychologist or psychiatrist with a special interest in somatic problems, even if patients do not wish to be referred for psychological treatment
- If you are concerned about a potential complaint, keep a detailed record of consultations, including any requests for investigations and the medical reasons for not ordering them. Repeated investigations that are not medically indicated can be unhelpful in increasing a patient's illness concerns. If you are worried about possible litigation, discuss the situation with a colleague and ask him or her to review the notes

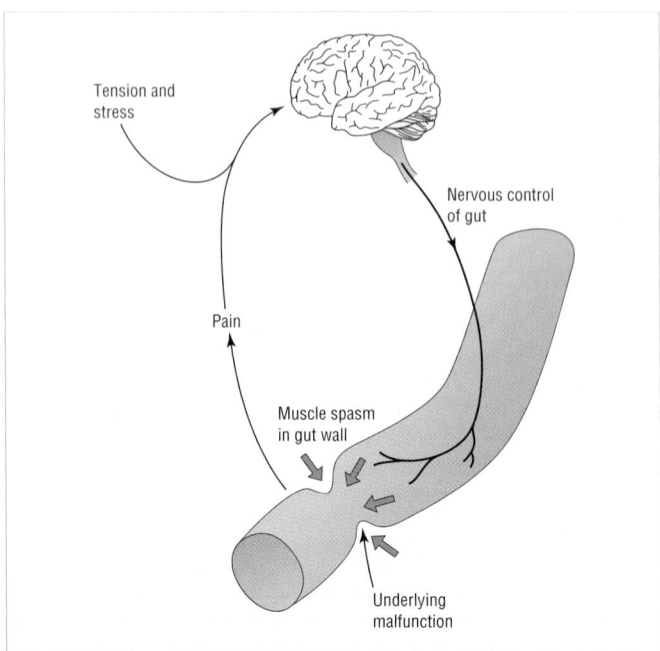

Explanation of how physiological and psychological factors combine to produce abdominal pain

---

Management of chronic functional abdominal pain
- Set the agenda
- Provide unambiguous information about findings
- Time planning: a longer planned session may save time in long run
- Identify psychosocial factors
- Set limits for investigations
- Encourage patient to take responsibility
- Don't treat what patient doesn't have

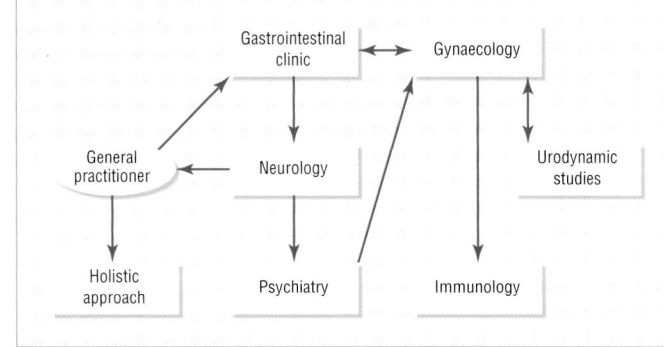

"Referral matrix" that can develop when managing a patient with chronic functional abdominal pain

---

Helpful patient organisations
- International Foundation for Functional Gastrointestinal Disorders. www.iffgd.org/
- IBS Network. http://homepages.uel.ac.uk/C.P.Dancey/ibs.html

- The aim of treatment should be to improve patients' symptoms and functioning rather than to abolish them. Although some patients may remain chronically disabled despite treatment, appropriate and consistent management can prevent deterioration and protect patients from unnecessary surgery.

Referral for psychological treatment

For patients who have not responded to initial management, four different kinds of psychological treatment have been evaluated in FGID. They are cognitive therapies, behavioural therapies, interpersonal therapies, and hypnosis. Each therapy has a different mechanism of action, but they have the common aims of reducing symptoms and improving functioning. Most treatments are delivered on a one to one basis, once weekly, over a period of two to four months.

Although most trials indicate a positive outcome for psychological treatment, many have methodological flaws and further studies are required before definitive recommendations about treatment can be given. The most convincing evidence for the efficacy of specific psychological treatments is for patients with chronic or refractory abdominal symptoms. However, there may also be an important role for earlier intervention in order to prevent such long term difficulties.

Psychological treatments are not always available. As in any other specialty, therapists need to have experience of treating chronic abdominal pain or chronic bowel disorders to develop and retain competence. Psychological services based in primary care are an option for patients with mild to moderate symptoms, but counsellors are unlikely to develop the expertise to enable them to treat patients with severe or refractory abdominal symptoms. Similarly, referral to a psychiatrist or psychologist who is more used to managing severe mental illness is unlikely to be fruitful. Dedicated medical liaison services with experience of somatic problems are more likely to be effective. If these do not exist consideration should be given to establishing a hospital based psychological medicine service.

The diagram of a biopsychosocial model for functional abdominal pain is adapted from Drossman DA et al, *Gut* 1999;45(suppl):II25-30.

Psychological treatments
Cognitive therapy
- Modifies patients' maladaptive beliefs about their pain and symptoms
- Encourages associated behaviour changes
- Patients keep diaries to monitor pain and other symptoms, associated thoughts, and behaviour
- As therapy progresses, it may be possible to identify underlying beliefs or fears about pain that drive preoccupation and worry
- Therapeutic work directed at activating three change mechanisms:
  1 Rational self analysis or self understanding (patients explore idiosyncratic beliefs and fears and connect these to their pain)
  2 Decentring (patients gain distance from their selves by identifying their self talk and labelling it)
  3 Experiential disconfirmation (patients challenge their fears or irrational beliefs through planned behavioural experiments)

Behavioural therapies
- Focus on changing behaviour; they do not address motives or fears
- Patterns that reinforce abnormal behaviour are identified and reversed
- Activity is gradually increased, particularly for functional activities such as social recreation and physical exercise
- Pain behaviours are ignored and activity related behaviours are reinforced
- Patients usually receive educational packages to increase their understanding of the condition
- Anxiety management strategies often included in treatment
- Biofeedback can be used to teach patients to reduce tension in affected muscles and to promote relaxation as a coping strategy

Interpersonal therapies
- Focus on resolving difficulties in interpersonal relationships that underlie or exacerbate abdominal symptoms
- Key problem areas include unresolved grief or loss, role transitions, and relationship discord
- Initial focus is on the patient's abdominal symptoms, which are explored in great detail
- Emotional distress and abnormal feeling states arising from or linked to physical symptoms are identified
- Key problem areas in relationships and their link to physical and psychological symptoms are understood
- Maladaptive relationship patterns, which may have developed after key childhood experiences (such as sexual abuse) are identified
- Solutions to interpersonal difficulties are tested out in therapy and implemented in real world

Hypnosis
- Directed at general relaxation
- Hypnosis is induced using an arm levitation technique, which is followed by deepening procedures
- General positive comments about health and wellbeing are made
- Patients are asked to place their hand on abdomen, feel a sense of warmth, and relate this to asserting control over gut function
- This is reinforced with visualisation (if patient has ability to do this)
- Sessions are concluded with positive, ego strengthening suggestions
- After third session patients are given a tape for daily autohypnosis

Further reading
- Thompson WG, Heaton KW, Smyth GT, Smyth C. Irritable bowel syndrome in general practice: prevalence, characteristics, and referral. *Gut* 2000;46:78-82
- Drossman DA, Creed FH, Fava GA, Olden KW, Patrick DL, Toner BB, et al. Psychosocial aspects of the functional gastrointestinal disorders. *Gastroenterol Int* 1995.1995:8:47-90
- Jailwala J, Imperiale TF, Kroenke K. Pharmacologic treatment of the irritable bowel syndrome: a systematic review of randomized, controlled trials. *Ann Intern Med* 2000;133:135-47
- Akehusrt R, Kaltenthaler E. Treatment of irritable bowel syndrome: a review of randomized controlled trials. *Gut* 2001;48:272
- Bytzer P. H$_2$ receptor antagonists and prokinetics in dyspepsia: a critical review. *Gut* 2002;50(suppl IV):58-62

Evidence based summary
- Treating functional gastrointestinal disorders with antidepressants is effective even in the absence of depression
- Although several psychological treatments show promise in treating functional bowel disorders, no trial has yet provided unequivocal evidence of effectiveness

Jackson J, O'Malley PG, Tomkins G, Balden E, Santoro J, Kroenke K. Treatment of functional gastrointestinal disorders with antidepressant medications: a meta-analysis. *Am J Med* 2000;108:65-72

Talley NJ, Owen BKO, Boyce P, Paterson K. Psychological treatments for irritable bowel syndrome: a critique of controlled treatment trials. *Am J Gastroenterol* 1996;91:277-86

13 Chest pain

Christopher Bass, Richard Mayou

Chest pain is one of the commonest reasons for consultation in primary care. Chest pain is usually mild and transient, but further management is required in some cases. These are of two main types—acute severe pain and persistent pain associated with distress and functional limitation. Acute central chest pain accounts for 20-30% of emergency medical admissions. Chronic chest pain is the commonest reason for referral to cardiac outpatient clinics.

Management of chest pain

The improved diagnosis and early treatment of ischaemic heart disease have not been accompanied by similar advances either in the delivery of long term rehabilitation of patients with ischaemic heart disease or in the management of non-cardiac causes of chest pain. Since at least half of those referred to cardiac outpatient clinics and about two thirds of emergency admissions have a non-cardiac cause for their chest pain, there is a pressing need to address this problem.

Primary care

Primary care doctors have a major responsibility for the continuing care of patients with angina and those with chronic non-cardiac chest pain, as well as a role in secondary prevention. They therefore need good communication with specialist cardiac services and access to appropriate resources, including psychological treatments.

Patients with a low risk of coronary disease (such as young women with no cardiac risk factors and atypical pain) do not usually need cardiac investigation. Some, however, especially those with chest pain who have a family history of heart disease or other risk factors, may need investigation. In such cases it is important that the possibility of a non-cardiac cause of the chest pain is explained before referral. If investigation reveals no cardiac cause for the pain patients need their worries to be fully discussed, need advice about coping with symptoms, and should be encouraged to maintain activity.

Patients with an intermediate or high risk (such as middle aged male smokers) often require investigations even if the chest pain is "not typical" of ischaemic pain. This will usually be achieved by referral to a cardiology outpatient clinic or to an emergency assessment service. When referring patients in whom the cause of chest pain is uncertain it is important to avoid giving them the impression that the diagnosis of ischaemic heart disease is already established (such as by prescribing anti-anginal drugs). This is because, if patients come to believe that they have ischaemic heart disease, such beliefs can be difficult to change even if they are subsequently disproved by investigation.

Secondary care

The best way to organise emergency care remains uncertain. A long wait for specialist investigations such as angiography is likely to increase anxiety and disability, as has been shown in patients waiting for coronary artery surgery. Quicker access to assessment (such as by rapid access clinics and observation units) can be helpful but needs to be accompanied by a greater emphasis on aftercare for all patients assessed, not only those who have had infarction or are undergoing cardiac surgery.

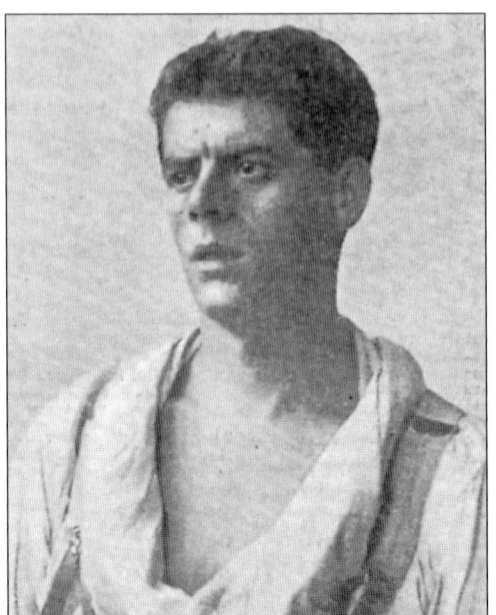

British soldier admitted for observation with the diagnosis of "disordered action of the heart"—a post-combat syndrome in the first world war characterised by rapid heartbeat, shortness of breath, fatigue, and dizziness. (From Lewis T. The tolerance of physical exertion, as shown by soldiers suffering from so-called 'irritable heart.' *BMJ* 1918;i:363-5)

Assessment and management of chest pain in primary care

- History of pain, other symptoms and risk factors
- If at high risk of heart disease, refer for specialist assessment
- If at low risk:
  Identify non-cardiac causes
  Give a positive explanation
  Advise how to cope with symptoms and return to normal activity
  Discuss worries
  Offer review if symptoms are persistent

Clinical priorities in managing patients with chest pain

Primary care
- Recognise and refer possible heart disease
- Reassure minor chest pain
- Basic treatment of persistent non-cardiac pain
- Reassess chronic pain as required, monitor and coordinate continuing care
- Advise on secondary prevention need

Hospital emergency care
- Immediate diagnosis and treatment plus initiating continuing care of angina
- Make a positive diagnosis; reassure if non-cardiac and arrange follow up to determine investigation and treatment needs
- Full and rapid communication with primary care

Cardiac outpatient care
- Initiate immediate and continuing care of angina
- Reassure and advise if non-cardiac; plan treatment or review

Other specialist care
- Cardiac rehabilitation or aftercare
- Psychological or psychiatric referral

Types of chest pain

Angina
The English national service framework for coronary heart disease recognises that patients' beliefs, attitudes, emotions, and behaviour are powerful determinants of clinical outcomes and suggests not only routine psychosocial assessment but also the integration of psychological approaches into cardiac rehabilitation programmes. Self help behavioural treatment programmes have also been shown to be of benefit. The general principles of treatment described below for non-cardiac chest pain are also applicable to angina.

Myocardial infarction and depression
About one in six patients who have a myocardial infarction develop major depression. The occurrence of depression has been found to be independently associated with poor outcome, including poor quality of life, increased heart disease, and probably increased mortality. There is some evidence that those who have the severest heart disease are at greatest risk of an adverse outcome attributable to depression. It is in just these patients that depression is most likely to be missed because both doctor and patient understandably focus their attention on the heart disease and its treatment, rather than on psychological factors.

Myocardial infarction, angina, and non-cardiac chest pain
Patients who have had a myocardial infarction or who have proved angina often report other chest pains that are clearly non-cardiac. Inevitably, they tend to misinterpret these symptoms as evidence of heart disease. The consequence is often greater disability and distress and a high and inappropriate use of medical care.

Non-cardiac chest pain
Fewer than half of the patients referred to emergency departments and cardiac outpatient clinics have heart disease. Over two thirds of these continue to be disabled by symptoms in the long term, and many also remain dissatisfied with their medical care. Some continue to take cardiac drugs and to attend emergency departments, primary care, and outpatient clinics. Hence, although these patients have a good outcome in terms of mortality, they suffer considerable morbidity.

It is desirable to make an early and confident diagnosis of non-cardiac chest pain because appropriate management of this condition in primary care can reduce subsequent morbidity.

Causes of non-cardiac chest pain
Explanations in terms of a single cause are rarely helpful. Instead, the cause is often best understood as an interaction of biological, psychological, and social factors. In many cases there is an interaction between normal or abnormal physiological processes (such as extrasystoles, oesophageal spasm or reflux, and costochondral discomfort), psychological factors (such as how somatic sensations are perceived, interpreted, and acted on), and the behaviour and reactions of other people, including doctors.

Establishing a positive diagnosis of non-cardiac chest pain

The key to establishing a positive diagnosis of non-cardiac chest pain, both in primary care and cardiac clinics, is, first, to consider the pattern of chest pain symptoms and, second, to seek evidence for non-cardiac causes.

Main components of cardiac rehabilitation treatment programme for patients with myocardial infarctions
- Provide education about heart attacks and secondary prevention and correct misconceptions
- Agree and record goals for exercise, return to work, and everyday activities; provide copies for patients, medical notes, and primary care
- Offer home exercise programme or community group exercise, or both
- Routine early review of symptoms, activity, and progress with rehabilitation and secondary prevention goals
- Menu of specific interventions, including stopping smoking, diet, and identification and treatment of psychological and behavioural difficulties

Non-cardiac pain in patients with diagnosis of angina
Diagnostic uncertainty may result in
- Non-cardiac pain being wrongly attributed to angina
- Increased antianginal medication
- Increased iatrogenic distress and disability
- Unnecessary investigations
- Unnecessary admissions and consultations

Common causes of non-cardiac chest pain
- Oesophageal disorders—Gastro-oesophageal reflux, oesophageal dysmotility
- Musculoskeletal—Costochondritis, increased muscular tension
- Referred pain from thoracic spine
- Hyperventilation
- Psychological—Panic attacks, depression

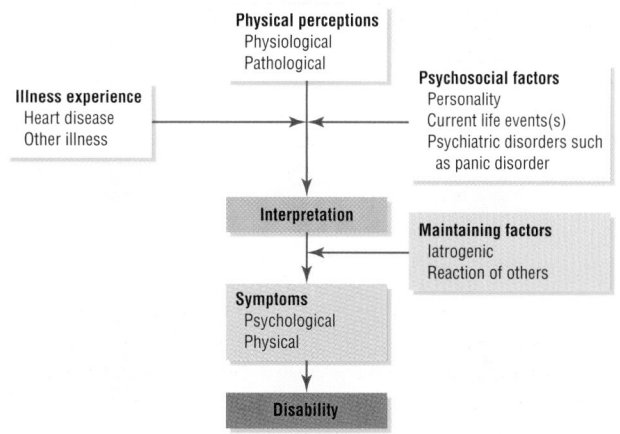

Interaction of biological, psychological, and social factors to cause non-cardiac chest pain and subsequent disability

Iatrogenic factors maintaining symptoms and disabilities
- Giving probable diagnosis of angina before investigation
- Immediate prescription of antianginal drugs without explanation of possible causes before investigation
- Lack of explanation for distressing and continuing symptoms
- Inconsistent or ambiguous information
- Reassurance contradicted by continued antianginal drugs or other indications of uncertainty
- Lack of communication with all involved in care leading to contradictory and conflicting advice

Quality of chest pain

Attempts to identify certain characteristics of chest pain that can help to establish a positive diagnosis of non-cardiac chest pain have been encouraging. For example, as few as three questions can differentiate patients with chest pain but normal coronary arteries from those with coronary heart disease.

Evidence for common non-cardiac causes

Oesophageal disorders are often associated with chest pain, but chest pain is poor correlated with objective oesophageal abnormalities. Symptomatic treatment (such as proton pump inhibitors) can be useful. Psychological issues may need addressing whether or not there is oesophageal pathology. Gastro-oesophageal reflux is an important cause of atypical chest pain, but there is no convincing evidence that such chest pain is often related to disturbances of oesophageal motility.

Emotional disorders—Only a minority of patients who present to family doctors with non-cardiac chest pain are suffering from conspicuous anxiety or depressive disorders. The rate of such disorders is, however, higher among those referred for specialist assessment in cardiac clinics, especially those who undergo angiography and are shown to have normal coronary arteries. It is important to seek evidence of (*a*) the key symptoms of depression (which include hopelessness; lack of interest, pleasure, and concentration; poor sleep; and irritability as well as low mood) and (*b*) an association of the chest pain with anxiety and panic attacks.

Patients' beliefs and worries

Even if no definite psychiatric diagnosis can be made, it is essential to ask patients what goes through their mind when they experience chest pain.

Stressful life events

Distressing life events can precipitate not only anxiety and depressive disorders, but also functional symptoms such as chest pain. Events signifying loss, threat, and rejection are of particular importance. Open questions are most effective in eliciting these—such as: "Tell me about any changes or setbacks that occurred in the months before your chest pain began."

Treatment of non-cardiac pain

Early and effective intervention is crucial, but how can this best be provided? Because patients vary not only in the frequency and severity of symptoms and associated disability but also in their needs for explanation and treatment of their physical and psychological problems, management needs to be flexible.

Avoiding iatrogenic worries—A consultation for chest pain is inherently worrying. Inevitably, many patients assume that they have severe heart disease, which will have major adverse effects on their life. These concerns may be greatly increased by delays in investigation, by comments or behaviours by doctors, and by contradictory and inconsistent comments.

Symptomatic treatment—In some patients the pain is obviously musculoskeletal in origin and can be treated with non-steroidal anti-inflammatory drugs. Proton pump inhibitors provide effective relief from the symptoms typical of gastro-oesophageal reflux, even in those with an essentially normal oesophageal mucosa. In some cases oesophageal function testing may reveal a motility disorder or acid reflux unresponsive to first line drugs. These patients may require specialist gastroenterological referral.

Communication—Problems in the care of patients with chest pain often arise from failures in communication between primary and secondary care. Lack of information and contradictory or inconsistent advice makes it less likely that patients and their

---

Questions to differentiate patients with non-cardiac chest pain from those with coronary heart disease

Question	Response	
	Typical	Atypical
If you go up a hill (or other stressor) on 10 separate occasions on how many do you get the pain?	10/10	< 10/10
Of 10 pains in a row, how many occur at rest?	< 2/10	≥ 2/10
How many minutes does the pain usually last?	< 5	≥ 5

When answers to all three questions are "atypical" the chance of coronary disease is only 2% in patients aged < 55 years and 12% in those aged ≥ 55

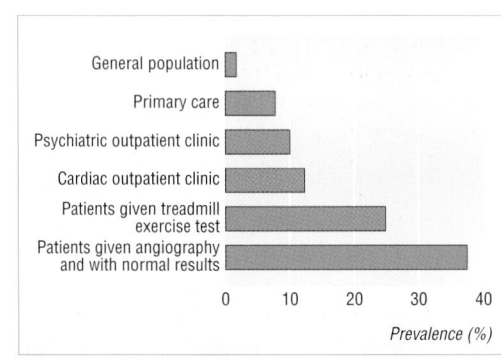

Prevalence of panic disorder in different medical settings

Screening questions for panic attacks

- In the past six months have you ever had a spell or an attack when you suddenly felt frightened, anxious, or very uneasy?
- In the past six months have you ever had a spell or an attack when for no reason your heart suddenly began to race, you felt faint, or you couldn't catch your breath?

If the answer is yes to either question then continue
- Obtain description
- Did any of these spells happen when you were not in danger or the centre of attention, such as in a crowd or when travelling?
- How many times have you had these spells in the past month?

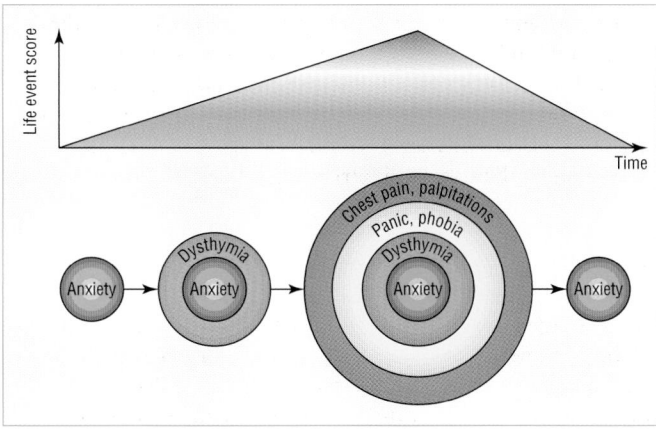

Life events and symptom reporting. Stress of adverse life events may result in increases in reporting of psychological and physical symptoms

---

Management of non-cardiac chest pain

General management
- Explanation of the diagnosis
- Reassurance that it is a real, common, and well recognised problem
- Advice on specific treatments
- Advice on behaviour—such as not avoiding exercise
- Discussion of concerns
- Provision of written information
- Involvement of relatives
- Follow up to review

Specialist treatments
- Cognitive behaviour therapy
- Antidepressant drugs
- Psychosocial intervention for associated psychological, family, and social difficulties

families will gain a clear understanding of the diagnosis and of treatment plans. The increasing use of computerised exchange of key information may reduce this problem, although it remains important to ensure that the information is passed on to and understood by patients and relatives.

Effective reassurance—Those with mild or brief symptoms may improve after negative investigation and simple reassurance. Further hospital attendance may then be unnecessary. Others with more severe symptoms and illness concerns will benefit from a follow up visit four to six weeks after the cardiac clinic visit (or emergency room visit), which allows time for more discussion and explanation. This may be with either a cardiac nurse in the cardiac clinic or a doctor in primary care. It also provides a valuable opportunity to identify patients with recurrent or persistent symptoms who may require further help.

Specialist treatments—Psychological and psychopharmacological treatment should be considered for patients with continuing symptoms and disability, especially if these are associated with abnormal health beliefs, depressed mood, panic attacks, or other symptoms such as fatigue or palpitations. Both cognitive behaviour therapy and selective serotonin reuptake inhibitors have been shown to be effective. Tricyclic antidepressants are helpful in reducing reports of pain in patients with chest pain and normal coronary arteries, especially if there are accompanying depressive symptoms.

Organising care

Because of the heterogeneity of the needs of patients who present with chest pain, we propose a "stepped" approach to management. A cardiologist working in a busy outpatient clinic may require access to additional resources if he or she is to provide adequate management for large numbers of patients with angina or non-cardiac chest pain. One way of doing this is to employ a specialist cardiac nurse who has received additional training in the management of these problems. The nurse can provide patient education, simple psychological intervention, and routine follow up in a separate part of the cardiac outpatient clinic. For those patients who require more specialist psychological care, it is important for the cardiac department (possibly the cardiac nurse) to collaborate with the local psychology or liaison psychiatry service.

Conclusion

The management of coronary heart disease has received much attention in recent years, whereas non-cardiac chest pain has been relatively neglected. The structuring of cardiac care for both angina and non-cardiac chest pain to incorporate a greater focus on psychological aspects of medical management would be likely to produce considerable health gains.

The picture of a soldier with "disordered action of the heart" is reproduced with permission of Wellcome Trust. The box of questions to identify patients with non-cardiac chest pain is adapted from Cooke R et al, *Heart* 1997;78:142-6. The figure showing link between life events and range of psychological and physical complications is adapted from Tyrer P, *Lancet* 1985;i:685-8. The figure of stepped care for managing non-cardiac chest pain is adapted from Chambers J et al, *Heart* 2000;84:101-5.

Effective reassurance

- Accept reality of symptoms
- Give explanation of causes
- Explain that symptoms are common, well recognised, and have a good prognosis
- Understand patient's and family's beliefs and worries
- Plan and agree simple self help
- Provide written information and plans
- Offer to see patient's partner or other close relative
- Offer follow up if required

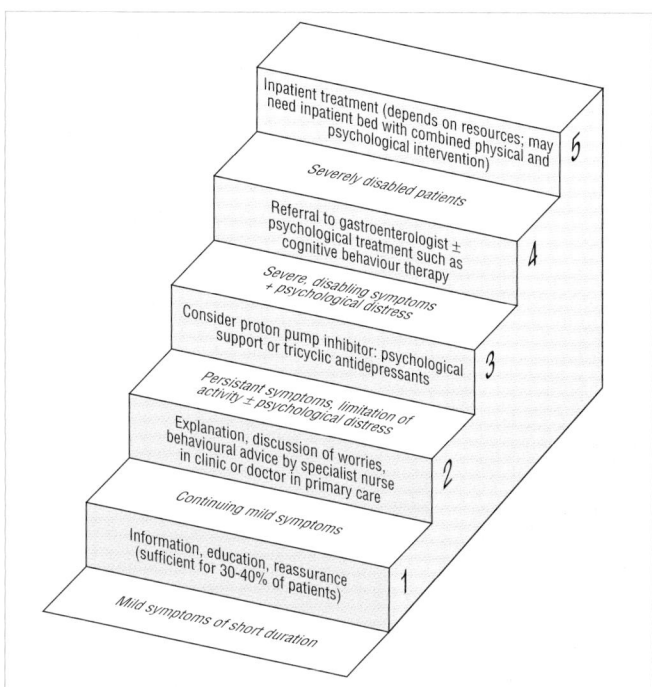

"Stepped" care in the management of non-cardiac chest pain

Evidence based summary

- Half of patients referred from general practice to a cardiac clinic with chest pain or palpitations do not have cardiac disease, but, despite the absence of disease, their symptoms tend to persist
- Psychological treatment and antidepressant drugs can be effective in treating non-cardiac chest pain

Mayou R, Bryant B, Forfar C, Clark D. Non-cardiac chest pain and benign palpitations in the cardiac clinic. *Br Heart J* 1994;72:548-53

Mayou R, Bryant B, Sanders D, Bass C, Klimes I, Forfar C. A controlled trial of cognitive behavioural therapy for non-cardiac chest pain. *Psychol Med* 1997; 27:21-31

Cannon RO 3rd, Quyyumi AA, Mincemoyer R, Stine AM, Gracely RH, Smith WB, et al. Imipramine in patients with chest pain despite normal coronary angiograms. *N Engl J Med* 1994;330:1411-7

Suggested reading

- Mayou RA, Bass C, Hart G, Tyndel S, Bryant B. Can clinical assessment of chest pain be made more therapeutic? *Q J Med* 2000;93:805-11
- Cooke R, Smeeton M, Chambers JB. Comparative study of chest pain characteristics in patients with normal and abnormal coronary angiograms. *Heart* 1997;78:142-6
- Creed F. The importance of depression following myocardial infarction. *Heart* 1999;82:406-8
- Jain D, Fluck D, Sayer JW, Ray S, Paul EA, Timmis AD. One-stop chest pain clinic can identify high cardiac risk. *J R Coll Physicians Lond* 1997;31:401-4
- Thompson DR, Lewin RJ. Management of the post-myocardial infarction patient: rehabilitation and cardiac neurosis. *Heart* 2000;84:101-5

14 Delirium

Tom Brown, Michael Boyle

Delirium is a common cause of disturbed behaviour in medically ill people and is often undetected and poorly managed. It is a condition at the interface of medicine and psychiatry that is all too often owned by neither. Although various terms have been used to describe it—including acute confusional state, acute brain syndrome, and acute organic reaction—delirium is the term used in the current psychiatric diagnostic classifications and the one we will use here.

Clinical features

Delirium usually develops over hours to days. Typically, the symptoms fluctuate and are worse at night. The fluctuation can be a diagnostic trap, with nurses or relatives reporting that patients had disturbed behaviour at night whereas doctors find patients lucid the next day.

Impaired cognitive functioning is central and affects memory, orientation, attention, and planning skills. Impaired consciousness, with a marked variability in alertness and in awareness of the environment is invariably present. A mistaken idea of the time of day, date, place, and identity of other people (disorientation) is common. Poor attention, and disturbed thought processes may be reflected in incoherent speech. This can make assessment difficult and highlights the need to obtain a history from a third party. Relatives or other informants may report a rapid and drastic decline from premorbid functioning that is useful in distinguishing delirium from dementia.

Disturbed perception is common and includes illusions (misperceptions) and hallucinations (false perceptions). Visual hallucinations are characteristic and strongly suggest delirium. However, hallucinations in auditory and other sensory modalities can also occur.

Delusions are typically fleeting, often persecutory and usually related to the disorientation. For example, an elderly person may believe that the year is 1944, that he or she is in a prisoner of war camp, and that the medical staff are the enemy. Such delusions can be the basis of aggressive behaviour,

Delirium can have a profound effect on affect and mood. A patient's affect can range from apathy and lack of interest to anxiety, perplexity, and fearfulness that may sometimes amount to terror. A casual assessment can result in an erroneous diagnosis of depression or anxiety disorder.

Disturbances of the sleep-wake cycle and activity are common. A behaviourally disturbed patient with night time agitation wandering around the ward is usually easy to recognise. However, presentations where a patient is hypo-alert and lethargic may go unrecognised.

Detection of delirium

Delirium often goes undiagnosed. Non-detection rates as high as 66% have been reported. Detection and diagnosis are important because of the associated morbidity and mortality: although most patients with delirium recover, some progress to stupor, coma, seizures, or death. Patients may die because of failure to treat the associated medical condition or from the associated behaviour—inactivity may cause pneumonia and decubital ulcers, and wandering may lead to fractures from falls.

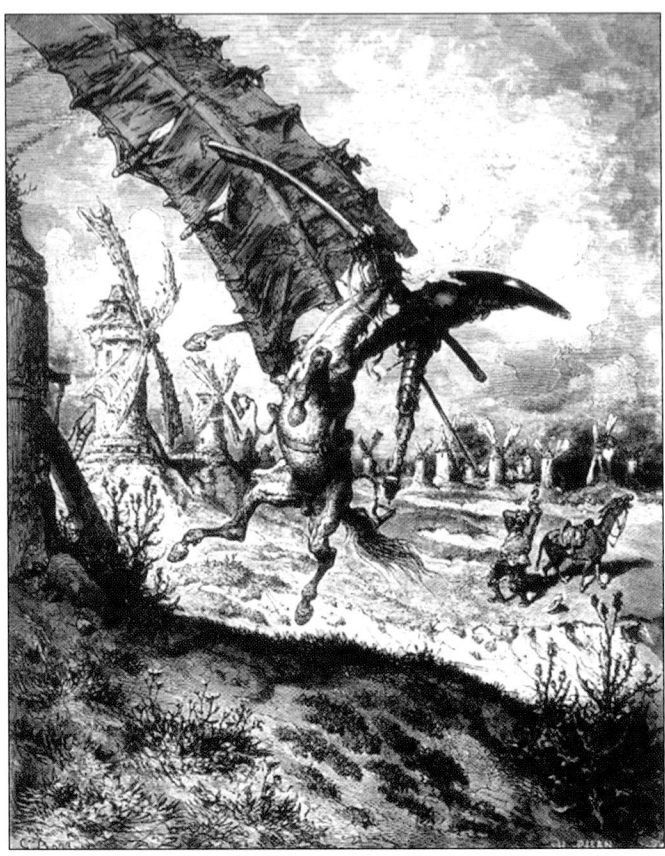

Sensory misperceptions, including hallucinations and illusions, are common in delirium. (*Don Quixote and the Windmill* by Gustave Doré, 1832-1883)

Diagnostic criteria for delirium*

- Disturbance in consciousness with reduced ability to focus, sustain, or shift attention
- Change in cognition (such as memory, disorientation, speech, disturbance) or development of perceptual disturbance not better accounted for by pre-existing or evolving dementia
- Disturbance develops over hours to days and fluctuates in severity

*Adapted from *Diagnostic and Statistical Manual of Mental Disorders*, 4th edition (DSM-IV)

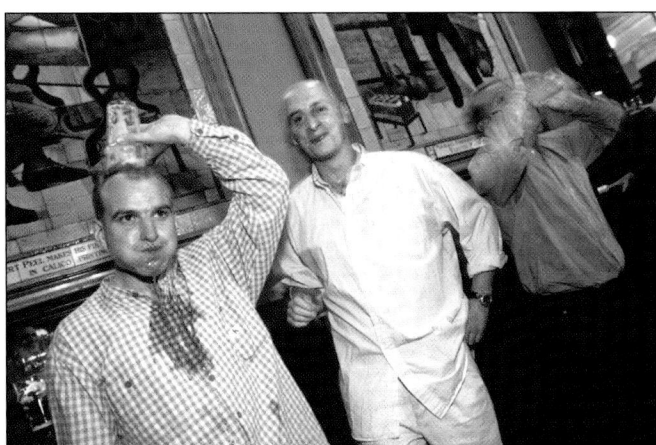

Alcohol addiction often goes undetected at the time of admission to hospital. All admitted patients should be asked about their alcohol consumption

Differential diagnosis

The main differential diagnosis of delirium is from a functional psychosis (such as schizophrenia and manic depression) and from dementia. Functional psychoses are not associated with obvious cognitive impairment, and visual hallucinations are more common in delirium. Dementia lacks the acute onset and markedly fluctuating course of delirium. Fleeting hallucinations and delusions are less common in dementia. It is important to note that delirium is commonly superimposed on a pre-existing dementia.

Prevalence

Most prevalence studies of delirium have been carried out in hospitalised medically ill patients, in whom the prevalence is about 25%. Most at risk are elderly patients, postoperative patients, and those who are terminally ill. The epidemiology of delirium in primary care and the community is unknown, but, with shorter length of stay in hospital and more surgery on a day case basis, it is likely to be increasingly common in the community and in residential care homes. It has been estimated that, among hospital inpatients with delirium, less than half have fully recovered by the time of discharge.

Aetiology

Delirium has a large number of possible causes. Many of these are life threatening, and delirium should therefore be regarded as a potential medical emergency. It is increasingly recognised that most patients have multiple causes for delirium, and consequently there may be several factors to be considered in diagnosis and management. Causes of delirium may be classified as

- Underlying general medical conditions and their treatment
- Substance use or withdrawal
- Of multiple aetiology
- Of unknown aetiology.

Prescribed drugs and acute infections are perhaps the commonest causes, particularly in elderly people. Prescribed drugs are implicated in up to 40% of cases and should always be considered as a cause. Many prescribed drugs can cause delirium, particularly those with anticholinergic properties, sedating drugs like benzodiazepines, and narcotic analgesics.

Withdrawal from alcohol or from sedative hypnotic drugs is a common cause of delirium in hospitalised patients separated from their usual supply of these substances. Delirium tremens is a form of delirium associated with alcohol withdrawal and requires special attention.

In addition to looking for precipitating causes of delirium, it is important to consider risk factors. These include age (with children and elderly people at particular risk), comorbid physical illness or dementia, and environmental factors such as visual or hearing impairment, social isolation, sensory deprivation, and being moved to a new environment.

Management

There are four main aspects to managing delirium:
- Identifying and treating the underlying causes
- Providing environmental and supportive measures
- Prescribing drugs aimed at managing symptoms
- Regular clinical review and follow up.

Good management of delirium goes beyond mere control of the most florid and obvious symptoms.

Distinguishing delirium from dementia

	Delirium	Dementia
Onset	Acute or subacute	Insidious
Course	Fluctuating, usually revolves over days to weeks	Progressive
Conscious level	Often impaired, can fluctuate rapidly	Clear until later stages
Cognitive defects	Poor short term memory, poor attention span	Poor short term memory, attention less affected until severe
Hallucinations	Common, especially visual	Often absent
Delusions	Fleeting, non-systematised	Often absent
Psychomotor activity	Increased, reduced, or unpredictable	Can be normal

Prevalence of delirium

Setting	% with delirium
Hospitalised medically ill patients*	10-30%
Hospitalised elderly patients	10-40%
Hospitalised cancer patients	25%
Hospitalised AIDS patients	30-40%
Terminally ill patients	80%

*High risk conditions and procedures include cardiotomy, hip surgery, transplant surgery, burns, renal dialysis, and lesions of the central nervous system

Causes of delirium due to underlying medical conditions

- Intoxication with drugs—Many drugs implicated especially anticholinergic agents, anticonvulsants, anti-parkinsonism agents, steroids, cimetidine, opiates, sedative hypnotics. Don't forget alcohol and illicit drugs
- Withdrawal syndromes—Alcohol, sedative hypnotics, barbiturates
- Metabolic causes
  Hypoxia, hypoglycaemia, hepatic, renal or pulmonary insufficiency
  Endocrinopathies (such as hypothyroidism, hyperthyroidism, hypopituitarism, hypoparathyroidism or hyperparathyroidism)
  Disorders of fluid and electrolyte balance
  Rare causes (such as porphyria, carcinoid syndrome)
- Infections
- Head trauma
- Epilepsy—Ictal, interictal, or postictal
- Neoplastic disease
- Vascular disorders
  Cerebrovascular (such as transient ischaemic attacks, thrombosis, embolism, migraine)
  Cardiovascular (such as myocardial infarction, cardiac failure)

Features of delirium tremens

- Associated with alcohol withdrawal
- Delirium with prominent anxiety and autonomic hyperactivity
- There may be associated metabolic disturbance and fits
- Chronic alcoholics are at risk of Wernicke's encephalopathy, in which delirium becomes complicated by ataxia and ophthalmoplegia. Urgent treatment with parenteral thiamine is required to prevent permanent memory damage

Making the diagnosis

Most patients with delirium are identified only because of marked behavioural disturbance. It would be preferable for all older patients to be screened for risk factors at admission to hospital. These would include substance misuse (particularly alcohol) and pre-existing cognitive impairment (assessed with the Hodkinson mental test or similar). Although such screening questions are part of the admission form in many hospitals, in our experience junior doctors seldom complete them. Once patients are admitted, minor episodes of confusion, behavioural disturbance, or increasing agitation should be taken seriously and investigated as appropriate. They should not be simply dismissed as "old age" or psychological reactions to hospitalisation.

Identifying and treating the cause

Delirium, by definition, is secondary to one or more underlying cause. Identifying such causes is often difficult, especially when patients are unable to give a coherent history or cooperate with physical examination. On occasions, it can be necessary to sedate a patient before conducting an adequate assessment. The interviewing of third parties is often helpful. Once a cause is found, appropriate treatment should be started without delay.

The environment

The aims of environmental interventions are, firstly, to create an environment that places minimum demands on a patient's impaired cognitive function and, secondly, to limit the risk of harm to the patient and others that may result from disturbed behaviour. Nursing should, as far as possible, be done by the same member of staff (preferably one trusted by the patient). This consistency should be supported with other strategies such as clear and if necessary repeated communication, adequate lighting, and the provision of clocks as aids to maintaining orientation. Visits from family and friends and provision of familiar objects from home can also be helpful. The correction of sensory impairments (such as by providing glasses or hearing aids) to help patients' grip on reality is sometimes overlooked.

It is also be important to minimise any risk to a delirious patient, other patients on the ward, and staff by ensuring that the patient is in a safe and separate area and that potentially dangerous objects are removed.

Drug treatment

Drug treatment of delirium should only be used when essential and then with care. This is because drugs such as antipsychotics and benzodiazepines can make the delirium worse and can exacerbate underlying causes (for example, benzodiazepines may worsen respiratory failure).

Antipsychotic drugs

Antipsychotics are the most commonly used drugs. Their onset of action is usually rapid, with improvement seen in hours to days. Haloperidol is often used because it has few anticholinergic side effects, minimal cardiovascular side effects, and no active metabolites. As it is a high potency drug it is less sedating than phenothiazines and therefore less likely to exacerbate delirium. It is, however, prone to causing parkinsonism, which may exacerbate a patient's tendency to fall. Low dose haloperidol (1-10 mg/day) is adequate for most patients. In severe behavioural disturbance haloperidol may be given intramuscularly or intravenously.

It is preferable to use a fixed dose that is frequently reviewed from the time of diagnosis rather than always giving the drug "as required" in response to disturbed behaviour. It is essential,

---

Hodkinson mental test

Score one point for each question answered correctly and give total score out of 10

Question

- Patient's age
- Time (to nearest hour)
- Address given, for recall at end of test (42 West Street)
- Name of hospital (or area of town if at home)
- Current year
- Patient's date of birth
- Current month
- Years of the first world war
- Name of monarch (or president)
- Count backwards from 20 to 1 (no errors allowed but may correct self)

Environmental and supportive measures in delirium

- Education of all who interact with patient (doctors, nurses, ancillary and portering staff, friends, family)
- Reality orientation techniques
  Firm clear communication—preferably by same member of staff
  Use of clocks and calendars
- Creating an environment that optimises stimulation (adequate lighting, reducing unnecessary noise, mobilising patient whenever possible)
- Correcting sensory impairments (providing hearing aids, glasses, etc)
- Ensuring adequate warmth and nutrition
- Making environment safe (removing objects with which patient could harm self or others)

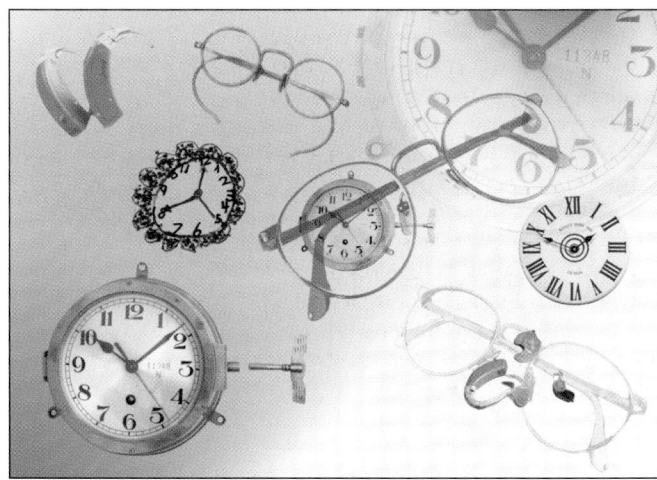

Simple measures to help orientation (such as glasses, hearing aids, and clocks) are effective in the management of delirium

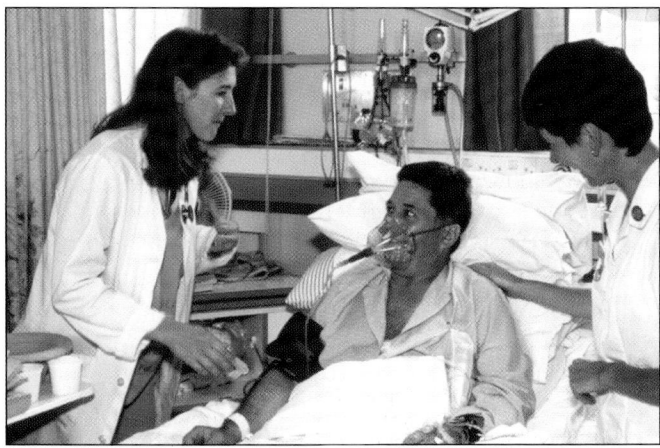

In postoperative patients judicious use of oxygen can treat delirium effectively

yet often forgotten, to monitor patients for both adequate response and unacceptable side effects. While a patient is in hospital this consists of at least a daily assessment of symptoms, level of sedation, and examination for extrapyramidal and other unwanted drug effects.

Preliminary experience with new antipsychotics suggest they may also be effective in delirium, but their advantages remain unestablished.

Benzodiazepines
Benzodiazepines are usually preferred when delirium is associated with withdrawal from alcohol or sedatives. They may also be used as an alternative or adjuvant to antipsychotics when these are ineffective or cause unacceptable side effects. Intravenous or intramuscular lorazepam may be given up to once every four hours. In patients with delirium due to hepatic insufficiency, lorazepam is preferred to haloperidol. Excessive sedation or respiratory depression from benzodiazepines is reversible with flumazenil.

Review
One of the most consistent failings in the management of delirium is lack of review. The acute symptoms are usually dealt with "out of hours" by junior staff and are forgotten by the next day. It is essential to review management of delirium and of the underlying causes for the duration of the hospital stay.

Patients' capacity and consent
Increasingly issues of capacity and informed consent may be raised in relation to the treatment of delirium. Urgent interventions needed to prevent serious deterioration or death or necessary in the interests of a patient's safety are deemed to be covered by common law in the United Kingdom. Although opinions differ, most agree that (*a*) if medical colleagues would deem a treatment appropriate and (*b*) if reasonable people would want the treatment themselves, then it can be given if urgently necessary.

Explaining the diagnosis
Effective management requires that not only the doctors and nurses caring for a patient understand the condition, but that the patient's family and friends appreciate the reasons for the dramatic change in the person's behaviour and that it is usually a reversible condition.

Aftercare
Many patients with delirium still have residual symptoms at the time of discharge from hospital. There is therefore a need for continued vigilance about medication, environmental change, and sensory problems during discharge planning and aftercare. Close liaison between hospital and primary care is an essential part of discharge planning.

Patients or their families will often need reassurance that an episode of delirium is not the start of an inevitable progression to dementia and that a full recovery can usually be expected. Delirious patients may erroneously be placed in long term care as "demented": decisions to place patients in care should be made only after an adequate assessment that differentiates delirium from dementia.

The picture of alcohol consumption is reproduced with permission of J Sutton and Rex Features. The picture of a patient receiving oxygen is reproduced with permission of Antonia Reeve and the Science Photo Library. The picture of pills is reproduced with permission of AJHD/DHD Photo Gallery

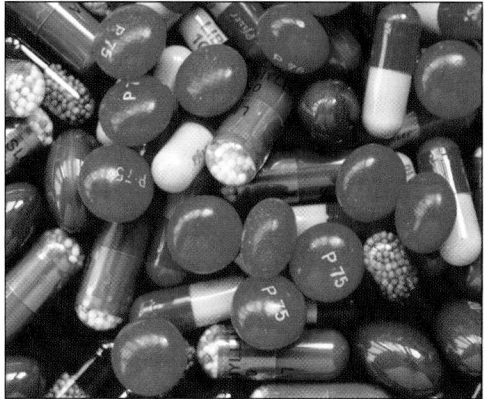
Excessive use of sedative drugs often causes more problems that it solves

Key medicolegal judgments about patients' capacity and consent (English Law)

Re c (mental patients: refusal of treatment) [1994] 1 WLR 290
An adult has the capacity to consent to or refuse treatment if he or she can
- Understand and retain the information relevant to the decision in question
- Believe that information
- Weigh the information in the balance to arrive at an informed choice

Re f (mental health sterilisation) v West Berkshire Health Authority (1989) 2 WLR 1025: (1989) All ER 673
"not only (1) must there be a necessity to act when it is not practicable to communicate with the assisted person but also (2) the action taken must be such as a reasonable person would in all circumstances take, acting in the best interests of the assisted person."
"Action properly taken to preserve life, health or wellbeing of the assisted person (which) may well transcend such measures as surgical operations or substantial treatment and may extend to include such humdrum matters as routine medical or dental treatment, even such simple care as dressing and undressing and putting to bed."

Evidence based summary
- A quarter of hospitalised elderly patients will have delirium
- Occurrence of delirium predicts poorer outcome and greater length of stay even after controlling for other variables, including severity of illness
- Positive identification and management of risk factors can reduce incidence and severity of delirium in elderly patients

Francis J, Martin D, Kapoor WN. A prospective study of delirium in hospitalized elderly. *JAMA* 1990;263:1097-101

O'Keeffe S, Lavan J. The prognostic significance of delirium in older hospital patients. *J Am Geriatr Soc* 1997;45:174-8

Cole MG, Primeau FJ, Elie LM. Delirium: prevention, treatment, and outcome studies. *J Geriatr Psychiatry Neurol* 1998;11:126-37

Further reading
- American Psychiatric Association. *Practice guideline for the treatment of patients with delirium.* Washington, DC: APA, 1999
- Meagher DS. Delirium—optimising management. *BMJ* 2001;322:144-9
- Meagher DS, O'Hanlon D, O'Mahony E, Casey PR. The use of environmental strategies and psychotropic medication in the management of delirium. *Br J Psychiatry* 1996;168:512-5
- Taylor D, Lewis S. Delirium. *J Neurol Neurosurg Psychiatry* 1993;56:742-51

Index

Page numbers in **bold** refer to figures in the text; those in *italics* refer to tables or boxed material

Index

Index